Contents

Diabetes Matters in Primary Care

Ruth Chambers

Jonathan Stead

and

Gill Wakley

Foreword by

Mike Pringle

Chair of Council

Royal College of General Practitioners

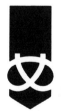

Staffordshire

UNIVERSITY

RADCLIFFE MEDICAL PRESS

Radcliffe Medical Press Ltd
18 Marcham Road
Abingdon
Oxon OX14 1AA
United Kingdom

www.radcliffe-oxford.com
The Radcliffe Medical Press electronic catalogue and online ordering facility.
Direct sales to anywhere in the world.

British Library Cataloguing in Publication Data

A catalogue record for this book is available from the British Library.

ISBN 1 85775 424 7

Typeset by Joshua Associates Ltd, Oxford
Printed and bound by TJ International Ltd, Padstow, Cornwall

Foreword

Nobody can doubt the importance of diabetes. One in 30 people have diabetes, and their life expectancy is greatly reduced – by about 20 years on average in type 1 diabetes and by 5–10 years in type 2. Diabetes is a risk factor for coronary heart disease, stroke, kidney failure, non-traumatic lower limb amputation and blindness. It is more common among some ethnic groups, the elderly and the obese, and is a major contributor to the health inequalities divide in the UK today.

Diabetes is becoming more common, partly due to the ageing of the population, the changing ethnic mix and the increase in obesity. The number of people with diabetes is expected to double in the next 20 years. It is often diagnosed late – up to 7 years late on average, when many individuals already have diabetic complications.

It is, most importantly, a chronic disease that is largely managed in primary care. Those people with diabetes who have complex needs – the young and those with complications – must be seen by secondary care-based teams. However, for most people their care is firmly focused in the community, with their GP, practice nurse, optician, dietitian and pharmacist.

Yet all of the evidence suggests that primary care for diabetes is highly variable and that, on the whole, it is failing people with diabetes, who receive little and often contradictory information. They do not feel in control of their diabetes, and they often do not receive the basic checks that they need. Moreover, poor control of blood sugar, blood pressure, lipids and lifestyle is all too often condoned and accepted.

This then is the core challenge – to improve the consistency and quality of clinical and psychological care, mainly through a patient-centred partnership approach. The National Service Framework will propagate this model and primary care trusts (PCTs) will be expected to deliver it on the ground in all sectors of the NHS. The mechanisms that the PCTs will use include commissioning, clinical governance, education, support and team development.

This is where this book comes in. There are many books on diabetes, but no others that explore so effectively the ways to deliver diabetic care in practice, combining clinical governance and personal and practice development planning. It is an excellent, lucid, up-to-date guide for GPs, nurses and all team members on how to meet the expectations of the National Service Framework for diabetes and to deliver what we all know is essential, namely a high-quality patient-focused service for those who live with diabetes.

Professor Mike Pringle
April 2001

About the authors

Ruth Chambers has been a GP for 20 years and is currently the Professor of Primary Care Development at Staffordshire University. Her service work has included a period as a clinical assistant in diabetes. Ruth has designed and organised many types of educational initiatives, including distance-learning programmes. Recently she has developed a keen interest in working with GPs, nurses and others in primary care around clinical governance and practice personal and professional development plans. She and Gill Wakley are producing a new series of books designed to help readers to draw up their own personal development plans or practice learning plans around important clinical topics such as diabetes.

Jonathan Stead has worked in a small rural general practice in Devon since 1981. He was first involved in diabetes research in 1986, working as a research fellow at the University of Exeter, and recruiting patients from practices for an early retinal screening project using mobile cameras in surgeries in Devon. As Chairman of Devon Medical Audit Advisory group, he has supervised a number of multi-practice diabetes audits, and more recently he has been involved in research into the management of the diabetic foot, and screening methods for the detection of diabetes. In 1993, he completed a research-based MPhil looking at practice nurse involvement in diabetes care in general practice. He has been associated with Diabetes UK for a number of years, and helped to develop their guidelines for the management of diabetes in primary care. He is currently the Clinical Governance Lead for Mid Devon Primary Care Group, the lead for the NHS R&D-funded Mid Devon Primary Care Research Group, and the primary care representative on the Local Diabetes Strategy Advisory Group. He works as a primary care affiliate with the NHS Clinical Governance Support Team.

Gill Wakley started in general practice in 1966, but transferred to community medicine shortly afterwards and then into public health. A desire for increased contact with patients caused a move back into general practice, together with community gynaecology, in 1978. She has been combining the two, in varying amounts, ever since.

Throughout she has been heavily involved in learning and teaching. She was in a training general practice, became an instructing doctor and a regional assessor in family planning, and was until recently a Senior Clinical Lecturer with the Primary Care Department at Keele University, Staffordshire. Like Ruth, she has run all types of educational initiatives and activities, from individual mentoring and instruction to small-group work, plenary lectures, distance-learning programmes, workshops and courses for a wide range of health professionals and lay people.

Acknowledgements

We have drawn heavily on the chapter on diabetes published in the *Health Care Needs Assessment* series.[1] This book individualises previous texts about continuing professional development[2] and clinical governance[3] setting them in the context of diabetes.

[1] Williams R and Farra H (2001) Diabetes mellitus. In: *Health Needs Assessment Series: the epidemiologically based needs assessment reviews*. Radcliffe Medical Press, Oxford (available online at http://hcna.radcliffe-online.com/diabframe.htm)
[2] Wakley G, Chambers R and Field S (2000) *Continuing Professional Development in Primary Care: making it happen*. Radcliffe Medical Press, Oxford.
[3] Chambers R and Wakley G (2000) *Making Clinical Governance Work for You*. Radcliffe Medical Press, Oxford.

Abbreviations

ACE	angiotensin-converting enzyme
ADA	American Diabetes Association
BDA	British Diabetic Association (now Diabetes UK)
DCCT	Diabetes Control and Complications Trial
DVLA	Driver and Vehicle Licensing Agency
HImP	health improvement programme
ICD	International Classification of Diseases
ICP	integrated care pathway
IFG	impaired fasting glycaemia
IGT	impaired glucose tolerance
LDSAG	Local Diabetes Services Advisory Group
LHG	local health group
NSF	National Service Framework
OGTT	oral glucose tolerance test
PCG	primary care group
PCO	primary care organisation
PCT	primary care trust
RCT	randomised controlled trial
SMR	standard mortality rate
SWOT	strengths, weaknesses, opportunities and threats
UKPDS	United Kingdom Prospective Diabetes Study
WHO	World Health Organization

Introduction

The material in this book sets out how learning more about diabetes mellitus and reviewing current practice can be incorporated into your personal development plan. You need to develop a dual focus on improving the clinical management of diabetes and increasing the efficiency of the working environment in the general practice. Practice team members should work together to direct their individual learning plans to form their practice personal and professional development plan. This should complement the business plan of the practice or primary care group/trust in England, the local health group in Wales or their equivalent bodies in the rest of the UK (all termed primary care organisations or PCOs hereafter).

The reason for focusing on diabetes is that it is a common disease, and much of the ensuing morbidity and premature mortality of diabetes in the UK is preventable. Over a million people in the UK have diabetes, the majority of whom have insulin-resistant type 2 (*see* Box 2.3), and three-quarters of them are looked after solely in primary care. Many people with diabetes do not comply with their treatment or lifestyle advice. The additional workload for NHS staff pursuing best practice, collaborative working and training has resource implications. Added to these are the costs of new medications and investigations. Your personal development plan should allow you to learn how to provide the care expected of you to address the goals and milestones set out in the National Service Framework (NSF) for diabetes.[1]

The NSFs for England incorporate integrated packages of care and give a clinical focus for strategic development of health services. NSFs should improve standards and the quality of care and reduce variations in services.[2] The national standards set out in the NSF for diabetes will be delivered locally through clinical governance and health improvement programmes. Delivery is underpinned by professional self-regulation, research and development into effective interventions, and human resources programmes. The Centre for Health Improvement (CHI), the NHS Performance Framework and the NHS Patient Survey will monitor the standards. The NSFs have a strong patient focus, including provision of good information, opportunities for patients to participate in decision making, and more transparency about service quality and outcomes.

You may decide to allocate 50% of the time you intend to spend drawing up and applying a personal development plan in any one year on learning more about diabetes. That would leave space in your learning plan for other important topics such as mental health, coronary heart disease or cancer – whatever is a priority for you, your practice team and your patient population. There will be some overlap between topics. For example, you cannot consider a person with diabetes in isolation from their cardiovascular risk factors, and that means understanding and knowing how to prevent and manage cardiovascular problems, too.

The first chapter of the book describes how a clinical governance culture incorporates effective clinical management and well-organised working conditions. You should be able to demonstrate that you are fit to practise as an individual clinician or manager (best practice in the management of diabetes in this case) and that your working environment is fit to practise from. This section will be relevant to all readers, whether you are a clinician or a primary care manager, as it will enable you to understand more of the context within which you work and how your individual contribution fits into the whole picture of healthcare.

Thereafter, each chapter gradually builds up your knowledge base of diabetes so that you can bring yourself up to date with the most recent evidence for managing diabetes. There have been a great many changes in recommended best practice in the last few years, as major research has provided evidence about preventing and managing the complications of diabetes. We shall usually cite evidence from a review or compendium rather than the original literature, to simplify the text in this book.

The whole programme builds up to the generation of a personal development plan and a practice personal and professional development plan in Chapters 9 and 10. Interactive exercises at the end of each chapter give the reader an opportunity to assess their learning needs, review their performance or that of the practice organisation, and reflect on what improvements to make.

You should transfer information from these needs assessment exercises to the relevant slots in your personal development plan as an individual, or your practice personal and professional development plan if you are working as a team.[3] Adopt a wide-based approach to improving quality – think of how you are establishing a clinical governance culture in your own practice team through your timed action plans.

What should you do next?

Study the templates for a personal development plan or a practice personal and professional development plan (also termed 'practice learning plan') on pages 101–33. You will be filling these in as you go along. Decide whether you will be starting out on your personal development plan or working with colleagues on the practice learning plan. Everyone's personal development plans should mesh with the practice learning plan by the time they have finished drawing them up.

Make changes as a result – to your workplace, or to the equipment in your practice, or to the advice you give patients, or to the way in which you manage and investigate diabetes or its complications.

CHAPTER 1

Clinical governance and the management of diabetes

Diabetes mellitus is a metabolic disorder characterised by chronic hyperglycaemia with disturbances of carbohydrate, fat and protein metabolism. Blood glucose is raised as a result of insufficient insulin production, or because the insulin that is produced is less effective due to the presence of factors which oppose its action.[4,5]

Clinical governance involves doing anything and everything required to maximise the quality of health care or services, including those for people with diabetes.[6]

The Commission for Health Improvement (CHI) defines clinical governance as 'the framework through which NHS organisations and their staff are accountable for the quality of patient care'.[7]

The CHI's view of clinical governance includes:

- a patient-centred approach which treats patients with courtesy, involves them in decisions and keeps them informed
- an accountability for quality which ensures that clinical care is up to date in their practices
- ensuring high standards and safety
- a demonstrable improvement in patient services and care.

We should be able to use clinical governance to improve the detection and control of lifelong chronic conditions such as diabetes. Clinical governance is inclusive – making quality everyone's business, whether they are a doctor, a nurse or other health professional, a manager, a member of staff or a strategic planner. Good diabetes care relies on the multidisciplinary team to support the person with diabetes in self-managing their disease inasmuch as they are able to do so. Delivering best practice requires an adequate number of clinical staff who are up to date and relate well to their patients, and efficient systems and procedures that are patient friendly.

Components of clinical governance

The components of clinical governance are not new. However, bringing them together under the banner of clinical governance and introducing more explicit accountability for performance is a new style of working.

The following 14 themes are core components of professional and service development which together form a comprehensive approach to providing high quality healthcare services and clinical governance.[6] These are illustrated in Figure 1.1.

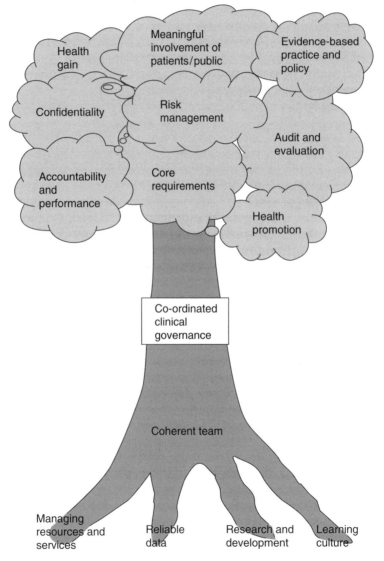

Figure 1.1: 'Routes' and branches of clinical governance.

If you interweave these 14 components into your individual and practice learning plans, you will have addressed the requirements for clinical governance at the same time.[3,6] The components are as follows:

1 learning culture – for patients and staff in the practice or primary care organisation or with secondary care
2 research and development culture – in the practice or throughout the health service
3 reliable and accurate data – in the practice, across the primary care organisation and across the NHS as a seamless whole
4 well-managed resources and services, as individuals, as a practice, across the NHS and in conjunction with other organisations
5 coherent team – well-integrated teams within a practice, including attached staff
6 meaningful involvement of patients and the public – including those with diabetes, those who care for them and the general population
7 health gain – from improving the health of staff and patients in a practice, between practices and in a primary care organisation
8 confidentiality – of information in consultations, in medical notes and between practitioners
9 evidence-based practice and policy – applying it in practice, in the district and across the NHS
10 accountability and performance – for standards, performance of individuals and the practice – to the public and those in authority
11 core requirements – good fit with skill mix and whether individuals are competent to do their jobs, communication, work-force numbers and morale at practice level
12 health promotion – for patients, the public, your staff and colleagues – both opportunistic and in general, or targeting those with most needs
13 audit and evaluation – for instance, of the extent to which individuals and primary care teams adhere to best practice in clinical management
14 risk management – being competent to spot those at risk, reducing risks and probability of ill health. This is particularly important in diabetes, where complications are common and have serious consequences.

The challenges to delivering clinical governance

Delivering high-quality healthcare with guaranteed minimum standards of care at all times is a major challenge. At present the quality of healthcare is patchy and variable. We are not very good at detecting under-performance and rectifying it at an early stage. The small number of clinicians who do under-perform exert a disproportionately large effect on the public's confidence. Causes of under-performance in an individual might be a result of a lack of knowledge or skills, poor attitudes or ill health or a lack of resources. A lack of management capability is nearly always a contributory reason for inadequate clinical services.

We need to understand why variation exists and explore ways of reducing inequalities. Variation in the quality of healthcare provided is common, whether it is between different practices in the same locality, between staff of the same discipline working in the same practice or unit, or between care given to some groups of the population rather than others. For instance, not all practices have written guidelines for referral of diabetes patients, some districts have systematic screening programmes for retinopathy whereas others do not, and some practices have easy access to a diabetic liaison nurse which others do not have.

Clinical governance offers a co-ordinated approach to overcoming these areas of risk.[7] The complex cultural change that will be required to deliver uniformly excellent care is immense. We need to develop measurable outcomes that professionals, patients and the public consider to be relevant and meaningful. Then we can assess the progress made, through implementing clinical governance, in the milestones and targets set out in the National Service Framework (NSF) for diabetes.

Box 1.1 Using diabetes as a tracer condition for a clinical governance programme[8]

Primary care groups in Newcastle upon Tyne developed indicators for the quality of diabetes care as an indicator of the quality of care that they provided in general. They set the following five parameters for the clinical governance programme:

- a disease register containing diabetic diagnoses
- treatment offered, including foot care and dietetic advice
- glycosylated haemoglobin (HbA_{1c}) results

- risk factors – blood pressure, cholesterol, smoking, alcohol intake, body mass index
- target organs affected – eyes, kidneys, heart, central nervous system, vascular changes.

The participating practices compared their results for the 1280 patients they had registered as having diabetes. A consultant diabetologist, the GP tutor and local general practitioners discussed the results at an educational meeting and agreed a plan to synchronise services between hospital, primary care and general practices. The health authority provided resources for improving care, education, training and clinical governance. A computerised template that includes the above five parameters will be adopted by the constituent practices to produce a shared database that will enable retrieval of information and recording of data.

Progress is being made with strengthening of the infrastructure and information systems across the primary care groups, and the establishment of a reliable surveillance programme for people with diabetes.

Learning culture

Education and training programmes should be relevant to service needs, whether at organisational or individual levels. Continuing professional development (CPD) programmes need to meet both the learning needs of individual health professionals and the wider service development needs of the NHS. You should no longer opt for CPD activities according to what you *want* to do, but rather according to what you *need* to do. Clinical governance underpins professional and service development.

Box 1.2

Individual personal development plans
will feed into a
practice-based personal and professional development plan
that will feed into
the practice's/primary care organisation's business plan
all of which are
underpinned by clinical governance.[3]

Multidisciplinary learning will boost close teamwork providing diabetic care.

Applying research and development in practice

The findings of the many thousands of research papers about diabetes that are published in reputable journals each year are rarely applied in practice. This is because few health professionals or managers read such journals regularly, and consequently they are not aware of the research findings. Most practice teams do not have a system for reviewing important research papers and translating that review into practical action. The primary care organisation might help by relaying important new evidence to its constituent practices or pharmacies, or to the general public. Improvements should result if working parties can agree on local disease templates (e.g. for diabetes) for recording data, and on making changes to working practices, provided that they are backed by resources.

Box 1.3
Incorporating research-based evidence into everyday practice should promote policies on effective working, improve quality and create a clinical governance culture.

Research increases our understanding of the causes and effects of diabetes as well as enabling the development of new treatments. For example, we understand more about insulin resistance, and the fact that it is probably caused by a combination of genetic and lifestyle factors, as a result of recent research. Decreased insulin sensitivity is inherited, but a high-fat diet, sedentary lifestyle and central obesity are implicated as causes, too. As insulin resistance is common, research and development of new insulin-sensitising drugs and other ways of reversing insulin resistance have the potential to make an impact on blood glucose control.

Reliable and accurate data

Clinicians, patients and administrators need access to reliable and accurate data. Set standards for a general practice to:

- keep records in chronological order
- summarise medical records within a specified time period for records of new patients
- review dates for checks on medication, with audit in place to monitor whether standards are adhered to, and to plan for under-performance if necessary
- use computers for diagnostic recording – agree Read codes for different diabetic classifications as in the NSF
- record information from external sources (hospital and other organisations) that is relevant to individual patients or practice.

Keep good written records of policies and audits that relate to diabetes in the practice. An inspection at any time should show what audits have been undertaken and when, the changes in practice organisation that followed, the extent of staff training undertaken, and the future programme of monitoring.

Well-managed resources and services

The things you need to achieve best practice should be in the right place at the right time and working correctly every time.
Set standards in your practice or workplace for:

- access to premises and availability of services for people with special needs (e.g. those with disability due to heart disease)
- provision of routine and urgent appointments (e.g. for those with diabetes)
- access to and provision for referral for investigation or treatment
- pro-active monitoring of chronic illness and disability
- alternatives to face-to-face consultations
- consultation length.

The primary care services to which the public requires access are information, advice, triage and treatment, continuity of care, personal care and other services.
Systems should be designed to prevent and detect errors. Therefore it is important to keep systems simple and sensible and to inform everyone how those systems operate, so that they are less likely to bypass a system or make errors. Sort out good systems for the follow-up of patients' diabetic clinical management.

Coherent teamwork

Teams do produce better patient care than single practitioners operating in a fragmented way. Effective teams make the most of the different contributions of individual clinical disciplines in delivering patient care. The characteristics of effective teams are:

• shared ownership of a common purpose
• clear goals for the contribution that each discipline makes
• open communication between team members
• opportunities for team members to enhance their skills.

A team approach helps different team members to adopt an evidence-based approach to patient care, by having to justify their approach to the rest of the team.[9] The different disciplines necessary for providing team-based diabetic care include the GP and practice nurse, non-clinical staff, optician or optometrist, dietitian, podiatrist and/or chiropodist and the community pharmacist, with help from other expert health professionals such as the diabetic specialist nurse and a hospital-based diabetologist.

Meaningful involvement of patients and the public

People use terms such as 'user' or 'consumer' to describe who they should be involving in giving feedback about the quality or type of healthcare on offer, or in planning future services. Patients or carers, non-users of services, the local community, a particular subgroup of the population or the general public will all have useful feedback and views (e.g. on your systems that inform people about the results of investigations or locating services closer to the patient).

The aims of user involvement and public participation include better outcomes of individual care and health of the population, more locally responsive services and greater ownership of health services.[10] Those planning the services should develop a better understanding of why and how local services need to be changed. You might want to consult the public and health professionals about the closure of a community hospital for example, without which those with chronic conditions such as diabetes may have to travel further for their care.

Box 1.4

Each local (e.g. district) planning group should consult with one or more relevant consumer groups so that customers can be given greater involvement in the development of their diabetic services.[11]

Health gain

The two general approaches to improving health are the 'population' approach, which focuses on measures to improve health through the community, and the 'high-risk' approach, which focuses on vulnerable individuals who are at high risk of the condition or hazard. We generally use a targeted approach to identify individuals whose diabetes was previously undiagnosed, rather than population screening.

The two approaches are not mutually exclusive, and they often need to be combined with legislation and community action. Health goals include:

- a good quality of life
- avoiding premature death
- equal opportunities for health.

Modifiable risk factors with potential health gains from reducing the risks of coronary heart disease in those people who have diabetes include:

- obesity
- lack of exercise
- smoking
- high lipid levels.

Several different interventions will usually be employed for a particular individual in order to optimise control of blood glucose, blood pressure and plasma lipids, and to help patients to lose weight and stop smoking.

Confidentiality

Confidentiality is a component of clinical governance that is often overlooked. Experienced health professionals and managers may assume that junior or new staff know all about confidentiality, and of course they may not. There are many difficult situations in the NHS where one person asks for information about another's medical condition (e.g. diabetic test results), where it is not clear-cut whether this information should be supplied or withheld, or even if it is acceptable to acknowledge that the person being enquired about is receiving care.

The Caldicott Committee Report describes the following principles of good practice to safeguard confidentiality when information is being used for non-clinical purposes.[12]

- Justify the purpose.
- Do not use patient-identifiable information unless it is absolutely necessary to do so.
- Use the minimum necessary patient-identifiable information.
- Access to patient-identifiable information should be on a strict need-to-know basis.
- Everyone with access to patient-identifiable information should be aware of his or her responsibilities.

Evidence-based culture – policy and practice

The key features determining whether or not local guidelines worked in one initiative[13] were as follows:

- there was multidisciplinary involvement when drawing them up
- a systematic review of the literature underpinned the guidelines, with graded recommendations for best practice linked to the evidence
- there was ownership at both national and local levels
- a local implementation plan ensured that the needs for resources, time, staff, education and training were foreseen, met and supported
- plans were made to sustain the guidelines – which were user friendly and could be modified to suit individual practitioners and patients.

Box 1.5

Two major studies have provided the evidence for optimising the control of blood glucose levels. These are the Diabetes Control and Complications Trial[14] and the United Kingdom Prospective Diabetes Study (UKPDS).[15] These studies show that the risk of developing microvascular complications with diabetes is substantially reduced at lower glycosylated haemoglobin (HbA_{1c}) levels in patients with type 1 and type 2 diabetes.

The hierarchy of evidence that is used to describe how scientifically a particular study was conducted, and therefore how reliable the conclusions are likely to be, varies between different reviews of published studies. There are several systems of grading evidence. A classification[16] that is often quoted gives the strength of evidence as shown in Box 1.6.

Box 1.6 Strength of evidence

Type 1:   Strong evidence from at least one systematic review of multiple well-designed randomised controlled trials (RCTs).

Type II: Strong evidence from at least one properly designed randomised controlled trial of appropriate size.

Type III: Evidence from well-designed trials without randomisation, single group pre–post, cohort, time-series or matched case–control studies.

Type IV: Evidence from well-designed non-experimental studies from more than one centre or research group.

Type V: The opinions of respected authorities, based on clinical evidence, descriptive studies or reports of expert committees.

Other categories of evidence are listed in the compendium of the best available evidence for effective healthcare, *Clinical Evidence*,[17] which is updated every six months, and is perhaps more useful to the health professional in everyday work (*see* Box 1.7).

Box 1.7

Beneficial: Interventions whose effectiveness has been shown by clear evidence from controlled trials.

Likely to be beneficial: Interventions for which effectiveness is less well established than for those listed under 'beneficial'.

Trade off between benefits and harms: Interventions for which clinicians and patients should weigh up the beneficial and harmful effects according to individual circumstances and priorities.

Unknown effectiveness:	Interventions for which there are currently insufficient data, or data of inadequate quality (this includes interventions that are widely accepted as beneficial but which have never been formally tested in RCTs, often because RCTs would be regarded as unethical).
Unlikely to be beneficial:	Interventions for which lack of effectiveness is less well established than for those listed under 'likely to be ineffective or harmful'.
Likely to be ineffective or harmful:	Interventions whose ineffectiveness or harmfulness has been demonstrated by clear evidence.

The Scottish Intercollegiate Guidelines Network (SIGN) has produced many guidelines relating to the management of diabetes, and their recommendations are based on similar evidence.[18–22]

Accountability and performance

Health professionals may not always realise that they are accountable to others from outside their own professions, especially if they are of self-employed status, as are GPs, pharmacists and optometrists. However, in fact they are accountable to:

- the general public
- the profession – to maintain the standards of knowledge and skills of the profession as a whole
- the government – and employer, who expect high standards of healthcare from the work-force.

Box 1.8

Health professionals who believe that they are not accountable to others may be reluctant to collect the evidence necessary to demonstrate that they are fit to practise, and that their working environment is fit to practise from. They may be reluctant to co-operate with central NHS requirements such as contributing to the local health improvement programme or working to the standards set out in the National Service Frameworks.

It is possible to identify and rectify under-performance at an early stage by, for example:

- regular appraisals (at least annually) linked to clinical governance and personal development plans as a process of regular supportive meetings between manager and staff member
- detecting those who have significant health problems, and referring them for help
- systematic audit that distinguishes individuals' performance from the overall performance of the practice team
- an open learning culture in which team members are discouraged from covering up colleagues' inadequacies, so that problems can be resolved at an early stage.

Clinicians may regard the performance assessment framework as a management tool that is not particularly relevant to their clinical practice. However, it does reinforce a clinical governance culture whereby good clinical management and organisational management have a symbiotic relationship.

Box 1.9

The NHS performance assessment framework has six components, namely health improvement, fair access, efficiency, effective delivery of appropriate care, user/carer experience and health outcomes.

Health promotion

People with diabetes will benefit if they are well informed about their condition and able to participate in making decisions about the management of the condition. Good information will help people with diabetes to make choices about their diet, smoking, physical activity and other health-related behaviour.

People with type 2 diabetes may mistakenly believe that their condition is trivial because they are asymptomatic when they are first identified as having diabetes. Therefore GPs and staff need to motivate them to comply with advice and treatment. One-third of patients with type 2 diabetes develop one or more clinical complications within ten years of diagnosis, including macrovascular disease (e.g. myocardial infarction, stroke), microvascular disease (e.g. retinopathy, nephropathy, neuropathy).

Box 1.10 Promotion of self-management of diabetes[23]

A review of the effectiveness of patient education about the management of type 2 diabetes reached the following conclusions.

- People with type 2 diabetes should be encouraged to be involved in their own care.
- Interventions should be appropriate to individual characteristics and take into account factors such as age, educational level and ethnic origin.
- Although many educational programmes produce desirable outcomes in the short term and reduced HbA_{1c} levels, further research is needed to determine whether these improvements are sustained.

Audit and evaluation

Follow-up of patients with diabetes is critical in order to achieve as tight a control as possible of blood glucose and blood pressure, whatever the type of diabetes. Audit will be key to checking that patients adhere to their treatment and professionals work according to best practice.

Box 1.11

Audit was used to show that establishing a weekly diabetic clinic in a rural practice improved the care of those 620 patients with diabetes, some of whom had previously been managed by shared care arrangements with a hospital 20 miles away. The clinic was staffed by a diabetic specialist twice a month, a diabetic nurse, a chiropodist, a dietitian and a retinal diabetic photography service, as well as practice staff. Attendance has risen from 72% to over 94%. HbA_{1c}, serum cholesterol, serum triglycerides and diastolic blood pressure levels improved, whilst body mass index remained unchanged. The GPs running the service calculate that the GP-based clinic is cost-effective, and they estimate that the savings to the primary care group are in the region of £25 000 per year.[24]

Core requirements

You cannot deliver clinical governance without well-trained and competent staff, the right skill mix of staff, a safe and comfortable working environment and the provision of cost-effective care. There is accumulating evidence that managing diabetes according to best practice is cost-effective,[24, 25] but research is still needed to investigate the relative cost-effectiveness of different methods of screening.[26]

A clinical governance culture addresses the recent challenges[2] in relation to the following:

- partnership – working together across the NHS to ensure the best possible care
- performance – acting to review and deliver higher standards of healthcare
- the professions and wider workforce – breaking down barriers between different disciplines (e.g. through multidisciplinary teamwork between GPs and nurses with pharmacists and optometrists)
- patient care – access, convenient services, and empowerment to take a full part in decision making about their own medical care and in planning and providing health services in general
- prevention – promoting healthy living across all sections of society, and tackling variations in care.

Risk management

People may underestimate relative risks as applied to themselves and their own behaviour. For example, many smokers accept the relationship between smoking tobacco and disease, but do not believe that they personally are at risk. People usually have a reasonable idea of the *relative risks* of various activities and behaviours, although their personal estimates of the *magnitude* of risks tend to be biased – small probabilities are often over-estimated, and high probabilities are often under-estimated.[27]

Risk management in general practice mainly centres on assessing the probability that potential or actual hazards will give rise to harm. Consider how bad the risk is, how likely the risk is, when the risk will occur, if ever, and how certain you are of estimates about the risks. This applies equally whether the risk is an environmental or organisational risk in the practice, or a clinical risk.

Good practice means understanding and managing risk – both clinical and organisational aspects. Undertaking audit more systematically will reduce the risks of omission. Common areas of risk in providing healthcare services include the following:[27]

- out-of-date clinical practice
- lack of continuity of care
- poor communication
- mistakes in patient care
- patient complaints
- financial risk – insufficient resources
- reputation
- staff morale.

Communicating and managing risks with patients on an individual basis depends on finding ways to explain those risks and elicit people's values and preferences. They can then make decisions themselves either to take risks or to choose between alternatives that involve different risks and benefits.

Having a good patient complaint system should reduce the risk of a recurrence of the event which originally triggered the complaint.

Reducing blood glucose and blood pressure levels to near normal reduces the risk of developing microvascular complications of diabetes, such as retinopathy. It is the actual reductions in blood glucose and blood pressure that are important, rather than the particular antihypertensive and hypoglycaemic medication that is used. Treating hypertension is at least as important as treating hyperglycaemia in the prevention of long-term complications.

Reflection exercise

Exercise 1

Review and plan your clinical management of diabetes. Think how you might integrate the 14 components of clinical governance into your personal development plan or your practice personal and professional development plan. Examples are given for each component listed below. Complete this yourself from your own perspective.

- *Establishing a learning culture:* e.g. informal discussion about diabetes guidelines between GPs, nurses and the local optometrist.
- *Managing resources and services:* e.g. review the roles and responsibilities for managing diabetic care of members of the practice team and attached staff.
- *Establishing a research and development culture:* e.g. share findings in key research papers on best practice for managing type 2 diabetes among the practice team.
- *Reliable and accurate data:* e.g. keep electronic records (both individual and team) so that everyone uses the same Read codes and enters data consistently. Any audit exercises can be repeated next year and the results compared.
- *Evidence-based practice and policy:* e.g. update the evidence-based protocol for type 2 diabetes.
- *Confidentiality:* e.g. review to ensure that everyone is adhering to an agreed code of practice for giving results or advice at the reception desk.
- *Health gain:* e.g. target those patients with diabetes for particular efforts with regard to reducing their risk factors for coronary heart disease.
- *Coherent team:* e.g. communicate new systems for screening for diabetes or related complications to the rest of the team.
- *Audit and evaluation:* e.g. undertake an audit and act on the findings to improve the quality of diabetic care.
- *Meaningful involvement of patients and the public:* e.g. listen to and act on the comments of those patients with diabetes about the care and services that you are providing.
- *Health promotion:* e.g. obtain or write literature promoting physical activity via local walks.
- *Risk management:* e.g. establish systems and procedures to identify, analyse and control clinical risks such as those arising from careless repeat-prescribing practices.
- *Accountability and performance:* e.g. keep good records of patients with diabetes to demonstrate best practice in the prevention of complications and clinical management.
- *Core requirements:* e.g. agree roles and responsibilities in the team, such as nurse referral to GPs; train receptionists to act in a crisis situation.

Now that you have completed this interactive reflection exercise, transfer the information to the empty template of the personal development plan on pages 101–10 if you are working on your own learning plan, or to the practice personal and professional development plan on pages 127–33 if you are working on a practice team learning plan. Don't forget to keep the evidence of your learning in your personal portfolio.

CHAPTER 2

Defining diabetes mellitus

Definitions

Diabetes mellitus is characterised by a raised blood glucose concentration (hyperglycaemia) due to either insufficient insulin or the presence of factors that oppose its action.[28] It is a chronic disease with substantial premature morbidity and mortality.

Box 2.1 World Health Organization definition of diabetes[4]

Diabetes mellitus describes a metabolic disorder of multiple aetiology characterised by chronic hyperglycaemia with disturbances of carbohydrate, fat and protein metabolism resulting from defects in insulin secretion, insulin action or both.

New diagnostic criteria

New guidelines for diagnosing and classifying diabetes came into effect in the UK in June 2000 (*see* Box 2.2). These World Health Organization guidelines[4] have been adopted by the Royal College of General Practitioners, the Royal College of Physicians, the Royal College of Nursing and the Association of Clinical Biochemists in consultation with Diabetes UK.[29]

Lowering the diagnostic threshold means that a greater number of people have been labelled as having diabetes – probably around 10% more who were previously on the borderline are now classified as being diabetic.

New *risk categories* have also been introduced. These are as follows.

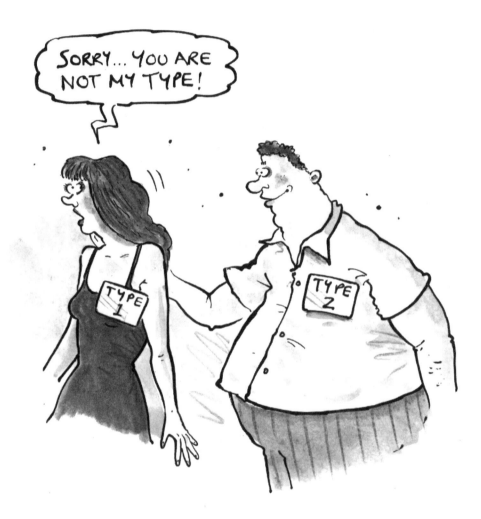

- Impaired glucose tolerance (IGT) is a state of impaired glucose regulation. This category indicates a risk for cardiovascular disease and future diabetes.

  Fasting plasma glucose < 7.0 mmol/L.

  Oral glucose tolerance test 2-hour value ≥ 7.8 mmol/L but < 11.1 mmol/L.

- Impaired fasting glycaemia (IFG) occurs in individuals who have fasting glucose levels above the normal range but below those diagnostic of diabetes. Individuals in this category are at risk of future diabetes. They should have an oral glucose tolerance test to exclude the diagnosis of diabetes, and should be strongly advised about adopting a less risky lifestyle – that is, to lose weight if they are overweight or obese, stop smoking, eat a well-balanced diet and take exercise as appropriate. Thus they should be encouraged to 'eat less and walk more'.

  Fasting plasma glucose > 6.1 mmol/L but < 7.0 mmol/L.

- Gestational diabetes now includes the categories of 'gestational impaired glucose tolerance' and 'gestational diabetes mellitus'.

Box 2.2 New diagnostic levels for diabetes mellitus[29]

With symptoms (polyuria, thirst, unexplained weight loss) plus

- a random venous plasma glucose concentration of > 11.0 mmol/L (whole blood equivalent is > 9.5 mmol/L)

or

- a fasting venous plasma glucose concentration of ≥ 7.0 mmol/L (whole blood equivalent is ≥ 6.1 mmol/L)

or

- a 2-hour venous plasma glucose concentration of > 11.0 mmol/L, 2 hours after administering 75 g of anhydrous glucose in an oral glucose tolerance test.

Without symptoms

- Diagnosis must not be based on a single glucose determination. Do a confirmatory test – at least one venous plasma glucose result on another day with a value in the diabetic range. This can be either a fasting or random sample, or from a 2-hour oral glucose tolerance test. If fasting or random values are not diagnostic, the 2-hour value after an oral glucose load should be used as the definitive test.

There are marked differences in threshold levels between venous plasma glucose and whole blood glucose (*see* Box 2.2). Patients usually have their blood glucose measured from a sample of whole blood in general practice. A blood glucose meter gives readings on samples of whole blood that are around 15% lower than those for venous plasma glucose. A whole blood sample which is sent to the hospital laboratory is reported as the plasma glucose.

A different approach should be taken with children. They usually present with severe symptoms and it is acceptable to make the diagnosis on the basis of a single raised blood glucose result. Refer such a child urgently to a paediatric diabetes team.

There are four sub-categories of diabetes:

1   type 1
2   type 2
3   gestational
4   other specific types (e.g. drug-induced).

The older terms 'insulin-dependent diabetes mellitus' and 'non-insulin-dependent diabetes mellitus' have been replaced by the categories type 1 and type 2 diabetes, respectively. This reflects their aetiology as well as the fact that people with *any* form of diabetes may require insulin treatment at some stage of their disease to improve the control of their blood glucose levels.

Box 2.3 provides more information about the differences between the various categories.

Box 2.3 Aetiological classification of diabetes mellitus[5]

Type 1 diabetes: β-cell destruction, usually leading to absolute insulin deficiency.

Type 2 diabetes: ranges from predominantly insulin resistance with a relative insulin deficiency to a predominantly secretory defect with insulin resistance.

Gestational diabetes mellitus

Other specific types:
- genetic defects in β-cell function
- genetic defects in insulin action
- diseases of the pancreas (e.g. pancreatitis)
- endocrinopathies (e.g. acromegaly)
- drug- or chemical-induced diabetes (e.g. caused by thiazides, steroids, thyroxine)

- infections (e.g. congenital rubella)
- uncommon forms of immune-mediated diabetes (e.g. due to anti-insulin antibodies)
- other genetic syndromes sometimes associated with diabetes (e.g. Down's syndrome).

Type 1

Type 1 diabetes encompasses diabetes due to pancreatic β-cell destruction or an auto-immune process. However, some forms of type 1 diabetes have no known aetiology.

Diagnosis of type 1 diabetes is usually straightforward if there are one or more of the classical symptoms of diabetes – thirst, polyuria, malaise and weight loss – taken together with a positive test for glucose in the urine or a raised blood glucose level.

Diabetes in children and adolescents usually presents with severe symptoms, although sometimes the symptoms may be less severe and require the additional confirmation of a fasting blood glucose or an oral glucose tolerance test. Various factors increase a child's risk of developing type 1 diabetes. These include intrauterine exposure to viral infections such as rubella or enterovirus, being the firstborn, and a high maternal age. The higher the maternal age at birth, the younger the age of onset of type 1 diabetes in the child. The inverse relationship between maternal age at delivery and the risk of diabetes was found to be equivalent to a 25% increase in risk for each 5-year rise in maternal age in one study.[30]

Type 2

The early symptoms of type 2 diabetes, such as tiredness, blurred vision, increasing thirst, weight loss and passing urine more often, may initially be attributed by the affected person to the effects of getting older. Because of this delay in presenting, half of those patients who are newly diagnosed may already have early signs of complications.

Type 2 diabetes may be caused by defects in insulin secretion, and usually by resistance to insulin. Type 2 diabetes is more common with older age, obesity, in various ethnic subgroups and families, and in individuals who take little physical exercise. The majority of people with type 2 diabetes are obese. Obesity itself causes or aggravates insulin resistance. A genetic component has been implicated in various forms of diabetes – as autosomal–dominant gene patterns and associated abnormalities of insulin action. Some genetic conditions, such as Down's syndrome, have an increased tendency to diabetes mellitus.

Insulin resistance distinguishes between type 2 and type 1 diabetes. Insulin resistance occurs when the body fails to respond to its own normally circulating insulin so that there is less of a blood-glucose-lowering effect. At first the body compensates by producing more insulin from the pancreas. However, less insulin is eventually produced as the β-cells of the pancreas become exhausted. A person with type 2 diabetes typically has reduced insulin secretion coupled with insulin resistance in the liver, adipose tissue and skeletal muscle, leading to a loss of control of blood glucose.

One cause of insulin resistance is thought to be the accumulation of surplus fat around the abdomen in preference to other parts of the body. The genetic make-up of people who are prone to insulin resistance encourages them to store surplus energy as abdominal fat rather than glycogen in skeletal muscle. This 'apple'-shaped human form is more likely to have a risk of early death from heart disease than a 'pear'-shaped form. Avoiding obesity and being physically active reduce the risks and effects of insulin resistance.

Gestational diabetes

Gestational diabetes affects 2–4% of pregnancies with a 'carbohydrate intolerance of variable severity with onset or first recognition in pregnancy'[21]. Thus women who were already known to have diabetes before becoming pregnant do not have 'gestational diabetes' – they have 'diabetes mellitus and pregnancy'. Lowering of the renal threshold for glucose in pregnancy is common.

Women who are most at risk for gestational diabetes are: older women, those with a previous history of glucose intolerance or babies that are large for gestational age, those from high-risk ethnic groups, and any pregnant woman with high fasting or random blood glucose levels. Women with a history of gestational diabetes should be screened for a recurrence in any future pregnancy. About two-thirds of women with gestational diabetes develop diabetes (usually type 2) within the next 20 years. Maintaining their weight within normal levels throughout their adult life reduces the risk of diabetes developing.

How common is diabetes?

Around 2–3% of people of all ages in the UK have types 1 or 2 diabetes.[5] About 200 000 people are thought to have type 1 and more than a million have type 2 diabetes.[31] More than 95 000 new cases of type 2 diabetes are diagnosed each year in the UK. There are a further million adults in the UK who are thought to have type 2 diabetes which is as yet undiagnosed. The lifetime risk for a person living in the UK developing type 2 diabetes is probably higher than 10%.[31]

Box 2.4

Prevalence rates summarise the proportion of the population with the disease (in this case diabetes) during a defined period of time.

$$\text{Prevalence} = \frac{\text{number of existing cases}}{\text{size of population during a defined period of time}}.$$

Box 2.5

Incidence rates describe the proportion of the population that develops the disease (in this case diabetes) during a defined period of time.

$$\text{Incidence} = \frac{\text{number of new cases}}{\text{size of population during a defined period of time}}.$$

The incidence of diabetes in children in the UK is around 14 per 100 000 children aged 14 years or under per year. The prevalence of diabetes in children and young people under 20 years of age is currently 14.0 per 1000.

Adults of South Asian and African-Caribbean origin are two to four times more likely to have diabetes (mainly type 2). However, there is little difference in prevalence of diabetes between children from various ethnic groups. Up to 20% of Asians and African-Caribbean people aged over 25 years living in the UK may have type 2 diabetes.

The prevalence of diabetes mellitus increases with age. As many as one in ten older people in the UK may have type 2 diabetes.[31]

Box 2.6

In Southall in London, the rates of those known to have diabetes are five times higher in South Asians than in other adults.[31]

The National Health Survey for England[32] attempted to assess how common undiagnosed diabetes might be. Researchers interviewed and tested about 12 000 adults and found that the prevalence of self-reported diabetes was 3% in men and 1.8% in women (the overall prevalence for men and women combined was 2.4%). The prevalence of *undiagnosed* diabetes was estimated from those with a glycosylated haemoglobin concentration of 5.2% or more who did not report that they were known to have diabetes. The prevalence of previously undiagnosed diabetes was 1% in men and 1% in women. The researchers concluded that the prevalence of all diabetes in the UK, diagnosed and undiagnosed, was 4% in men and 2.8% in women, with an average of 3.4% in all adults.

Box 2.7 below gives some idea of how many patients present as new cases of diabetes each year. Box 2.8 shows the known prevalence in a Midlands practice with a patient population of 10 628.

Box 2.7 The frequency of diagnosis of new cases of all types of diabetes in adults in the UK[5]

Age group (years)	Frequency of diagnosis of new cases of diabetes (all types) per 10 000 people per year
15–24	2.5
25–34	4.5
35–44	8.0
45–54	18.0
55–64	35.0
65–74	46.0
75–84	37.0
≥ 85	37.0

The total prevalence of diabetes in the UK has been predicted to rise by 25% and 14% for males and females, respectively, from 1992 to 2010.[5] The anticipated rise is due to three factors, namely the ageing of the population, the increase in adult obesity which contributes to the increase in the number of people with type 2 diabetes, and the increasing incidence of type 1 diabetes in children. The rates are predicted to double every 20–30 years.[5]

Box 2.8 An example from practice: the prevalence of diabetes in the Milton practice in Stoke-on-Trent where the patient population is 10 628

| Age group (years) | Number of patients known to have diabetes | | | | Total |
| | Type 1 | | Type 2 | | |
	Male	Female	Male	Female	
5–16		3			
17–24	1	1			
25–34	6	2	1	2	
35–44	2	7	7	7	
45–54	8	3	17	13	
55–64	1	3	20	28	
65–74	4	2	46	46	
75–84	3		26	29	
85–89			3	6	
≤90				6	
Total	25	21	120	137	303 (2.9%)

Costs of diabetes in the UK

Diabetes and its complications currently account for almost 10% of all health service spending in the UK, or nearly £5 billion. The direct costs of diabetes include the costs of preventing, diagnosing, managing and treating the condition, including hospital costs and the costs of care provided by Social Services. The total direct costs for people with type 2 diabetes in the UK in 1998 were estimated to be £1.83 billion, or 3.4% of healthcare expenditure.[33]

Indirect costs result from the consequences of morbidity, disability and premature mortality, and the loss of productive output for society. Indirect costs are difficult to calculate, but they have been estimated to be at least as great as the direct costs.[5]

People with diabetes use hospital services more than those without diabetes. One estimate in 1997 was that 8.7% of acute-sector costs are spent on the care of patients with diabetes.[5] People with microvascular complications of diabetes cost 2.5 times more to the NHS than patients with diabetes without complications, and those with macrovascular complications such as heart disease cost 2.7 times as much.[34]

Patients with diabetes have a fourfold higher probability of undergoing a cardiac procedure[5]. The total cost of the hospital treatment of coronary heart disease in people with diabetes in the UK has been estimated to be £1.1 billion at 1994/95 prices,[5] and the annual cost of caring for people with type 2 diabetes has been put at £2 billion. A patient with type 2 diabetes who has complications is twice as likely to need a carer, and will cost Social Services up to four times as much, as a patient with type 2 diabetes without complications.[34]

Earlier diagnosis and tighter control of glycaemia and blood pressure should result in fewer patients with diabetes having serious complications. The resources invested in improved health surveillance, identifying people with diabetes earlier, and encouraging them to comply with best practice should be more than balanced by the cost savings from prevented complications, and these patients' enhanced well-being and ability to work.

Box 2.9

Preventive foot care has been shown to reduce the need for hospital admission for lower limb complications (in Australia), to reduce amputation rates (in the UK) and to reduce the cost of diabetic foot disease (in The Netherlands).[5]

The UK Prospective Diabetes Study (UKPDS) trial showed that effective control of blood pressure with ACE inhibitor or beta-blocker drugs in people with diabetes is cost-effective.[15,34] The additional resources required to achieve this control were recouped within the 10 years of the trial by the cost savings from fewer complications and from additional life years gained.

Intensive therapy to improve the control of blood pressure or control of hyperglycaemia is more costly than routine care, but there are significant reductions in direct healthcare costs and considerable benefits in the longer term.[11,35] An economic evaluation of the UKPDS trial assessed the cost benefits of intensive glycaemic control. Intensive blood glucose control in patients with type 2 diabetes increased the treatment costs by a mean of £695 per patient, but reduced the risk of complications by a mean of £957 per patient compared with conventional treatment.[35]

Reflection exercises

Exercise 2

Review your practice protocol for diabetes (if you have not got a practice protocol for managing diabetes, now is the time to write one; *see* Chapter 7 for more details) and what your practice team knows about diagnosis and definitions.

 (i) Have you updated the diagnostic thresholds already? Do so and consider the implications. There are probably a number of patients who were previously on the borderline and who will now be categorised as having diabetes.

 (ii) Do all of the practice team know and understand the new diagnostic criteria? Try asking them over coffee.

(iii) Have all of the practice team converted to describing diabetes mellitus as different 'types' rather than using the old terminology about insulin use? Observe what they write in the records when you see patients who have recently consulted your colleagues.

(iv) Are all practice team members who provide care for diabetes aware of the different diagnostic levels for blood glucose depending on whether plasma or whole blood is taken? Ask them about this.

Exercise 3

How many people have you identified as having diabetes by type in your practice population? How do the proportions compare with the National Health Survey for England[32] described in this chapter? Do you need to redouble your efforts to identify people with diabetes from among your patients?

 Ask your local public health department for any information they have about your patients with diabetes. If there is a district diabetes register with health outcomes recorded by secondary and primary care, you may obtain additional information about your patients and compare your detection rates with those of other practices.

> Now that you have completed these interactive reflection exercises, transfer the information to the relevant sections about justifying the view that diabetes is a priority, and about your learning needs, in the empty template on pages 110–10 if you are working on your own personal development plan, or to the practice personal and professional development plan on pages 127–33 if you are working on a practice team learning plan. Don't forget to keep the evidence of your learning in your personal portfolio.

CHAPTER 3

Screening for undiagnosed diabetes mellitus

By the time many of those individuals with type 2 diabetes are diagnosed they may already have complications from their diabetes that have insidiously occurred in direct response to high blood glucose levels over the preceding years. Thus there is potential here for screening. Debate continues about the relative merits of population screening or opportunistic screening of targeted groups of people at risk, because it is not clear whether population screening for undiagnosed diabetes is both clinically effective and cost-effective.

Box 3.1

Screening is 'the systematic application of a test or inquiry, to identify individuals at sufficient risk of a specific order to warrant further investigation or direct preventive action, amongst persons who have not sought medical attention on account of symptoms of that disorder'.[36]

The American Diabetes Association advocates three-yearly testing for diabetes in all adults aged 45 years or over, whereas screening for diabetes in the general population in the UK is not advocated at present.

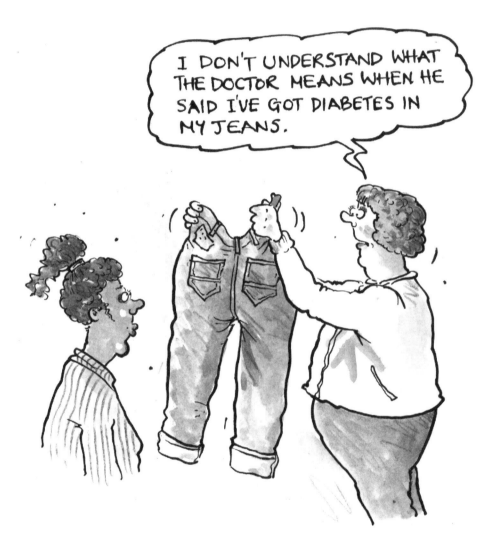

Specificity and sensitivity

> **Box 3.2**
>
> Sensitivity refers to the proportion of individuals with the target disorder (in this case diabetes) who test positive, too. Specificity refers to the proportion of individuals without the target disorder (in this case diabetes) who test negative for the disease.

Any screening programme has false positives and false negatives, which generate unwarranted worry and reassurance, respectively.

Population screening

Any population-based screening programme should fulfil the World Health Organization's criteria for screening. These are as follows.

- The disease or condition should be an important public health problem.
- There should be diagnostic procedures and adequate screening tests by which the disease or condition can be identified.
- There should be an effective treatment.

Box 3.3 below describes the results of population screening in Ipswich (the number of individuals who were diagnosed as having diabetes and the effort involved).

> **Box 3.3** Screening the general population for diabetes using a self-testing method[5]
>
> A total of 13 795 subjects in Ipswich who were aged between 45 and 70 years and not known to have diabetes were posted a urine testing strip with instructions and a result card. Of the 10 348 individuals (75%) who responded, 343 (3.3%) were found to have glycosuria, and diabetes was confirmed in 99 (30%) of the 330 subjects who attended for an oral glucose tolerance test (OGTT). A further 65 individuals had an OGTT result in the impaired glucose tolerance (IGT) range. Thus large-scale screening seemed to be possible and relatively cheap in terms of the cost of materials. However, around 140 people had to be contacted for each true positive case detected and the short- and long-term consequences of making these early diagnoses were not evaluated.

Opportunistic screening

Opportunistic screening or 'case finding' offers 'testing of apparently asymptomatic individuals not otherwise seeking medical care'.[37] The earlier that people with diabetes are identified, the more likelihood there is of preventing or delaying complications by good glycaemic control.

The symptoms of type 2 diabetes develop slowly over a period of years, so the initial symptoms may be vague. Over 75% of people who are at higher risk of diabetes, such as those described below, are unaware of their increased risk.

Diabetes UK recommends[38] that those in primary care use targeted screening to identify patients with diabetes by:

- screening all pregnant woman
- testing patients for diabetes if they report thirst, polyuria and weight loss, other urinary symptoms such as nocturia and urinary incontinence, recurrent infections, neuropathic symptoms such as pain, numbness and paraesthesia, or vague/unexplained symptoms such as lassitude
- considering an underlying diagnosis of diabetes in patients with hypertension, ischaemic heart disease, peripheral vascular disease or cerebrovascular disease.
- being more alert to the possibility of diabetes in the obese, people of Asian, African or African-Caribbean origin, people aged over 65 years, individuals with a family history of diabetes or cardiovascular disease, and women with a history of gestational diabetes or who have given birth to a baby weighing $> 4\,kg$.
- flagging the notes of people with a family history of diabetes or a personal history of gestational diabetes
- screening people at increased risk of diabetes every three years.

Screening for gestational diabetes[5]

Test the patient's urine for glycosuria at every antenatal visit. Organise timed random laboratory blood glucose measurements whenever glycosuria (1+ or more) is detected, at the booking visit and at 28 weeks' gestation.

A 75-g oral glucose tolerance test with laboratory blood glucose measurements should be carried out if the timed random blood glucose concentrations are > 6 mmol/L in the fasting state or 2 hours after food, or > 7 mmol/L within 2 hours of taking food.

Reflection exercise

Exercise 4

(i) Do you have a well-established screening programme targeted at high-risk patients in your practice? If not, draft guidelines or a protocol to be agreed with your practice team. If you do have such a programme, undertake an audit of 20 patients with hypertension who are not known to have diabetes, and see whether they have been screened for diabetes within the last three years. Are your records computerised with appropriate Read coding so that you can perform audits easily and randomly select patients from a disease register? If not, take 20 consecutive patients with hypertension as they consult you instead.

(ii) Visit a neighbouring practice and compare the way in which you screen your patients with their systems and procedures. Compare your practice protocols for the management of diabetes and hypertension while you are there. Look for gaps and refine your protocols accordingly.

Now that you have completed this interactive reflection exercise, transfer the information to the relevant section about your learning needs in the empty template on pages 101–10 if you are working on your own personal development plan, or to the practice personal and professional development plan on pages 127–33 if you are working on a practice team learning plan. Don't forget to keep the evidence of your learning in your personal portfolio.

CHAPTER 4

Complications

Macrovascular and microvascular complications are largely irreversible. Adults with diabetes are twice as likely to die each year as people without diabetes. Their annual mortality is about 5.4% and their life expectancy is reduced by an average of five to ten years.[22] A person with type 2 diabetes is two to four times more likely to suffer from heart disease, stroke and peripheral vascular disease than someone without diabetes.

Macrovascular complications of diabetes include cardiovascular disease, cerebrovascular disease (CVD) and peripheral vascular disease (PVD). Stroke or circulatory problems of the lower limbs result in ischaemic pain, ulceration, gangrene and amputation.

Coronary heart disease death rates are several times higher in people with diabetes than in those without the condition. Cardiovascular disease kills up to 75% of people with type 2 diabetes. The risk of coronary heart disease in people with diabetes cannot be explained by the presence of the classic risk factors for coronary heart disease – smoking, hypertension and raised serum lipid concentrations – diabetes seems to confer its own risk.[5]

Microvascular complications lead to retinopathy, nephropathy and neuropathy which occur either alone or in combination with each other.

Box 4.1 Vascular complications of diabetes

Macrovascular complications
   Coronary heart disease
   Cerebrovascular disease – stroke
   Peripheral vascular disease

Microvascular complications
   Retinopathy
   Nephropathy
   Neuropathy

The longer a person has diabetes, the more likely they are to develop complications. Coexisting risk factors such as hypertension, hyper-cholesterolaemia and cigarette smoking interact with diabetes to make complications more likely.

Table 4.1 describes the relative risks of various complications occurring in people with diabetes compared with individuals without diabetes.

Table 4.1 Risks of morbidity associated with all types of diabetes mellitus[22]

Complication	Relative risk*
Blindness	20
End-stage renal disease	25
Amputation	40
Myocardial infarction	2–5
Stroke	2–3

* Magnitude of risk compared with people without diabetes.

Mortality and morbidity from diabetes is higher in people from lower socio-economic groups, the unemployed, and in those who left full-time education at a young age.[5]

Microvascular complications

Retinopathy[20,26,39,40]

Diabetic retinopathy is a common and preventable cause of visual impairment and blindness.

About 13% of new cases of blindness in the UK among people aged 16–64 years are diabetes related.[33] Up to 40% of people with newly diagnosed type 2 diabetes have some degree of retinopathy, unlike those with type 1 diabetes, where significant retinopathy that would threaten the person's vision almost never occurs in the first five years after diagnosis or before puberty. Almost all individuals with type 1 diabetes and 60% of those with type 2 diabetes will have some form of retinopathy 15–20 years after diagnosis.

Box 4.2 Retinal signs of diabetic retinopathy

Classification of retinopathy	Signs
Background	Haemorrhages Micro-aneurysms Exudates
Pre-proliferative	Cotton-wool spots Venous changes Intra-retinal microvascular anomalies
Proliferative	New vessels Fibrovascular proliferation

Retinopathy is more likely to occur with longer duration of diabetes and poorer control of blood glucose and hypertension. The duration of diabetes is the most important factor that predicts whether retinopathy occurs and how severe it is. Both hypertension and cigarette smoking accelerate retinopathy.

Good glycaemic control can prevent the onset, slow down the progress and reduce the severity of diabetic retinopathy. About 10% of patients with background retinopathy progress to more severe retinopathy.[20]

Box 4.3

Tightening blood pressure control by 10 mmHg systolic and 5 mmHg diastolic over 8.4 years resulted in a 37% reduction in microvascular complications, including retinopathy, in one study.[5]

Hyperglycaemia causes a thickening of the basement membrane of retinal cells. Small blood vessels become blocked or leaky, causing oedema and then microvascular leakage and occlusion. Background retinopathy is due to red blood cells leaking and lipids being deposited on the retina to form micro-aneurysms, small blot haemorrhages and hard exudates. As the damage progresses, hard exudates may appear near the macula (exudative maculopathy), clusters of haemorrhages arise and macular oedema may occur, resulting in central visual loss.

The three characteristic signs of preproliferative retinopathy include 'cotton-wool spots', venous abnormalities and large haemorrhages. New fragile blood vessels start to proliferate and grow into the potential space between the retina and the vitreous humour. They form haphazardly on the peripheral retina and at the optic disc, and they bleed and scar if left untreated. A haemorrhage between the retina and vitreous humour is classically boat-shaped. A vitreous haemorrhage can cause a sudden burst of 'floaters' or complete blurring of vision. In advanced diabetic eye disease there is extensive fibrovascular proliferation, with the possibility of irreversible eye damage from retinal detachment as the fibrous tissue contracts and vitreous haemorrhage or thrombotic glaucoma occurs.

Box 4.4

Blindness is defined as visual acuity of $< 3/60$. Partial sight is defined as visual acuity of between 6/60 and 3/60 in the better eye.

Laser photocoagulation is effective in preventing blindness by arresting the progression of maculopathy and preventing further loss of vision, rather than restoring lost vision. Retinopathy is most amenable to treatment in the early stages, when there may be no symptoms of visual loss. New vessels will be abolished by treatment in 80% of patients with proliferative retinopathy. Continued follow-up and further photocoagulation can mean that the eye disease is stabilised or effectively cured. Laser treatment helps 50% of those with macular damage, too.

Box 4.5

Less than 50% of individuals with diabetes who received photocoagulation experienced severe visual loss or blindness, compared to untreated controls, in one study.[26]

The Driver and Vehicle Licensing Agency requires people who have had bilateral macular laser treatment to take a postoperative visual field test to determine whether they are fit to drive a car.

Aspirin and ticlopidine may reduce the rate of micro-aneurysm formation in early retinopathy, but these research findings are as yet unconfirmed.[39] Other drugs, such as growth-hormone antagonists, antihypertensive agents and somatostatin analogues, are under trial as treatments for proliferative retinopathy.

Cataracts are more common in people with diabetes. They tend to occur at an earlier age and have worse outcomes with surgical treatment than in non-diabetic patients. Macular degeneration and glaucoma are more common in people with diabetes, too.

Two-thirds of individuals who have proliferative diabetic retinopathy also have nephropathy. Those with retinopathy are significantly more likely to develop signs of renal disease than those without retinopathy.[23]

Screening for diabetic retinopathy[5,20,26]

Everyone aged over 12 years who has diabetes needs an annual screen for diabetic retinopathy.

Screening for retinopathy in individuals with diabetes fulfils all of the World Health Organization's criteria for a screening programme. American studies have demonstrated that preventing visual impairment in people with diabetes is cost-effective, as the costs of screening and subsequent treatment are lower than the costs of dealing with the blindness that would otherwise have resulted.

Systematic screening for diabetic retinopathy could prevent 260 new cases of blindness per year among people aged 70 years or under in England and Wales. Screening is patchy, and some areas do not have systematic screening programmes. A survey of 40% of screening programmes in England and Wales showed that fewer than half of the people known to have diabetes were included.

For every 100 patients with diabetes with treatable eye disease, 55 individuals could be expected to become blind or severely visually impaired within ten years if none of them were treated. However, if those 55 patients were detected and treated, only 13 individuals would be so affected.

Ophthalmologists and optometrists usually now use a slit-lamp biomicroscope and hand-held lens instead of a direct ophthalmoscope to gain a much wider field of view. Training improves the rate of detection of retinopathy.

Ophthalmoscopy and retinal photography can be combined for added benefits. Ophthalmoscopy allows examination of a wider field of the retina than is captured by photography. Retinal photography provides a lasting record of the extent of retinopathy, allowing comparisons over time as well as checks on the performance of the treating clinician. Studies have shown that ophthalmologists and optometrists are more accurate at diagnosing retinopathy using combined ophthalmoscopy and retinal photography compared with general practitioners, who were not as good at detecting retinopathy.

Box 4.6

In Shropshire, optometrists trained by the local diabetes service screened people with diabetes referred by general practitioners in their community-based clinics. A total of 8000 people have been screened, representing 90% of the target population. Ten per cent were referred to ophthalmologists and a fifth of these received laser treatment. Little difference was found between the accuracy of the reports from the optometrists and the results of retinal photography.[26]

The consensus is that annual screening for diabetic retinopathy by digital retinal photography with or without direct ophthalmoscopy is appropriate. Recommendations on how to organise such screening are listed in Box 4.7.

Box 4.7 Recommendations for screening for retinopathy[26]

- Screening should be provided for all people with diabetes who are not being treated for retinopathy.
- The screening service should be organised at a local level to cover all of the population of people with diabetes.
- Screening is effective if it is provided by accredited optometrists, reimbursed on a per capita basis, or by mobile retinal photography in various locations.
- There is insufficient evidence to allow specific recommendations to be made about the best methods of screening, which may vary according to local circumstances.
- Training should be provided for screeners.

Nephropathy[18,23]

Hyperglycaemia is associated with slow but progressive damage to the kidneys. The quantity of protein that is excreted in the urine increases as the renal disease becomes more severe.

Diabetic nephropathy is the most common single cause of end-stage renal failure among adults starting on renal replacement therapy.

People with type 2 diabetes are as susceptible to nephropathy as those with type 1 diabetes. People with type 1 or type 2 diabetes account for about a quarter of renal transplants. Two-thirds of patients with diabetes who have end-stage renal failure have type 1 diabetes, as those with type 2 are more likely to have died of cardiovascular complications before their renal disease reaches an end stage.

Box 4.8

People with diabetes who had proteinuria were followed up for 12 years in one study, to find that they had an eightfold (women) and fivefold (men) increased risk of death compared to those people with diabetes who did not have proteinuria.[23]

The three stages of diabetic nephropathy are as follows:

1 incipient nephropathy, when microalbuminuria is present, and the trace of protein present is not detectable by dipstick testing. Microalbuminuria predicts overt diabetic nephropathy, especially in patients with type 1 diabetes
2 overt disease with proteinuria, which takes about 5 to 15 years to develop
3 end-stage renal disease, which requires dialysis or renal transplantation.

About 25% of patients with type 2 diabetes develop microalbuminuria, and around 15% develop proteinuria over time. The UKPDS trial[15] found that 12% of patients with type 2 diabetes had microalbuminuria and 2% had proteinuria, when their diabetes was diagnosed. Box 4.9 shows the relevant incidence and prevalence rates.

Box 4.9 The prevalence of microalbuminuria, incidence of proteinuria and prevalence of proteinuria in people with diabetes[5]

Complication	Type 1 diabetes	Type 2 diabetes
Prevalence of microalbuminuria	10–25	15.0–25.0
Incidence of proteinuria	0.5–3.0	1.0–2.0
Prevalence of proteinuria	15.0–20.0	10.0–25.0

Prevalence rates are per 100 individuals with clinically diagnosed diabetes. Incidence rates are per 100 individuals with clinically diagnosed diabetes per year.

The main risk factors for nephropathy are hereditary susceptibility, hyperglycaemia and raised blood pressure. Advanced renal disease leads to increased blood pressure, and increased blood pressure in turn accelerates the development of diabetic renal disease.

People of Asian and African-Caribbean origin are susceptible to diabetic renal disease, and are six times more likely to be receiving treatment for end-stage renal failure than Caucasians with diabetes.

Screening for renal disease

The definition of microalbuminuria is 20–200 micrograms/minute in urine collected in patients at rest, or 30–300 micrograms/24 hours in a 24-hour sample. The SIGN guidelines suggest that it is more practical to use the first voided urine sample for screening purposes, rather than a timed collection over 24 hours.[18, 23]

Recommendations are as follows.

- The urine of patients with all types of diabetes should be tested at least annually for proteinuria and blood, and if the results of this test are negative, for microalbuminuria.[23]
- Diabetic patients with microalbuminuria should be re-tested within 6 to 12 weeks to confirm the presence of microalbuminuria.[18]
- Remember that urinary infection, poorly controlled diabetes, physical exercise, uncontrolled hypertension, cardiac failure, acute febrile illness, haematuria, menstruation and vaginal discharge may account for microalbuminuria, rather than its presence necessarily indicating renal disease.[18]
- Macroalbuminuria or overt proteinuria should be quantified by a 24-hour urine collection. Mid-stream urine samples, renal ultra-sonography, and measurement of immunoglobulins, autoantibodies and complement levels exclude other causes of proteinuria. A renal biopsy may confirm diabetic nephropathy or exclude non-diabetic renal disease.

Neuropathy

Diabetic neuropathies include both progressive and reversible types. Neuropathy is one of the commonest long-term complications of diabetes. The commonest type is a diffuse polyneuropathy which affects distal peripheral nerves in a symmetrical distribution. It mainly affects the feet and legs, gradually involving progressive sensory loss which includes reduced or absent ankle reflexes. Sometimes there is motor involvement with associated weakness and muscle wasting as well. People who have lost sensation in their feet are at risk from ill-fitting shoes or other trauma. Neuropathic foot ulceration may follow, which may lead to gangrene and amputation.

Symptoms range from severe burning or shooting pains to complete insensitivity to pain. There may be altered temperature sensation, hyperaesthesiae or paraesthesiae. Symptoms are usually worse in bed at night.

Around 7% of newly diagnosed patients with type 2 diabetes who are aged between 25 and 65 years have impaired sensation in the feet due to peripheral neuropathy. Neuropathy eventually affects 50% of all patients with type 2 diabetes, who are over 60 years of age.

Autonomic neuropathy is an irreversible progressive form that results from damage to both the parasympathetic and sympathetic nerves. The gastrointestinal, cardiovascular, genito-urinary and respiratory systems may be affected. Diarrhoea may be watery, nocturnal and intermittent. Postural hypotension may also be a problem.

Erectile dysfunction is often multifactorial and secondary to autonomic neuropathy, vascular insufficiency and psychogenic factors. Impotence is more common in people with diabetes, occurring in up to 50% of men over 50 years of age, compared with about 20% of non-diabetic men of similar age.[36] The presence of nocturnal erections may distinguish a psychogenic cause of erectile dysfunction from an organic cause, in which nocturnal erections may no longer occur.

Urinary retention occurs at a late stage in autonomic neuropathy.

Mononeuropathies are reversible and usually recover within 3–18 months depending on the type. Painful neuropathies affect one or both legs or the abdominal wall, and the pain is often severe and persistent. Diabetic amyotrophy produces pain and sometimes wasting in one or both thighs. Radiculopathy causes nerve root pain in almost any part of the body. Third and sixth cranial nerve palsies may also occur, presenting as a sudden onset of double vision.

Macrovascular complications

Coronary heart disease[5,15,22,40]

Coronary heart disease is the leading cause of death in people with all types of diabetes. In the UK Prospective Diabetes Study there were

70 times more cardiovascular deaths than deaths from microvascular complications.

The risk of coronary heart disease in people with type 2 diabetes is two to three times higher in men and four to five times higher in premenopausal women, compared with the corresponding risk in people without diabetes. Myocardial infarction is about two to three times more common in people with diabetes. Patients with diabetes who have an acute myocardial infarction are twice as likely to die as individuals without diabetes, while in hospital and at six months. People with diabetes who have a history of coronary heart disease have a very high risk of future macrovascular disease. It is important to be able to link up the coronary heart disease register in your practice with the diabetes register in order to identify these vulnerable individuals readily. This is difficult if the practice is not using Read codes based on the national minimum dataset.

Heart failure is five times more common in people with diabetes than in those without diabetes.

Other risk factors for coronary heart disease are additive. Diabetic patients who smoke have a higher mortality from coronary heart disease than do non-smokers.

One-third to one-half of middle-aged people with diabetes are hypertensive (34% of men aged 45–54 years, 40% of men aged 55–64 years, 44% of women aged 45–54 years old and 53% of women aged 55–64 years).

Hypertension and abnormal lipid levels are more common in individuals with both types of diabetes than in those without diabetes. Patients with type 2 diabetes have twice the mortality risk from coronary heart disease if they are hypertensive.

Box 4.10 Predictors of cardiovascular mortality[40]

Type 1 diabetes	*Type 2 diabetes*
Overt nephropathy	Presence of coronary heart disease
Hypertension	Overt proteinuria
Smoking	Higher levels of glycosylated haemoglobin
Microalbuminuria	Hypertension
Age	

Stroke[5]

Stroke accounts for about 15% of all deaths in people with diabetes.[32] The risk of atherothrombotic stroke is two to three times higher in people with diabetes, whilst the risks of haemorrhagic stroke and transient ischaemic attacks are similar to those in people without diabetes. As most strokes have an atherothrombotic cause, this is yet more bad news for those with diabetes. Strokes that occur in people with diabetes tend to be irreversible, and such patients have a higher death rate or more severe neurological damage.

Peripheral vascular disease[5]

Atherosclerosis in the coronary, cerebral and peripheral arteries is more common in individuals with diabetes than in people of the same age without diabetes. Insulin resistance accelerates atherosclerosis in patients with type 2 diabetes, mediated through hyperinsulinaemia, dyslipidaemia and hypertension. People with type 2 diabetes are more likely to have a risk-inducing lipid profile, with high total cholesterol, raised LDL-triglyceride and decreased HDL-cholesterol levels.

People with type 2 diabetes of all ages are more than twice as likely to develop peripheral vascular disease as those with type 1 diabetes. A quarter of those with type 2 diabetes develop peripheral vascular disease, whilst 12% of men and 5% of women with type 1 diabetes develop peripheral vascular disease.

Reflection exercises

Exercise 5

Undertake a significant event audit of a serious adverse condition that has occurred recently in someone with diabetes – for example, a patient with diabetes having a myocardial infarction or becoming blind. Look at the circumstances leading up to the event. Discuss the case as a practice team, looking to see whether you could have intervened more effectively at any time before the serious complication reached its final stage. Was the patient's diabetes well controlled? Could the management have been more effective?

Exercise 6

Undertake an audit of those patients with diabetes and coronary heart disease. Produce a list of all of these patients and note the type of diabetes.

(i) Have you recorded current smoking status in the last year?

(ii) Do you know which interventions for smoking cessation are most likely to be successful and for which patients with diabetes they are warranted?

(iii) Check the blood pressure, glycaemic control and cholesterol of these patients in the last year. Are these results within the recommended ranges (*see* Chapter 5)?

Exercise 7

First, ask 10 consecutive patients with diabetes who consult you to describe what risks they perceive they have of developing complications of diabetes. Are their perspectives realistic?

Second, ask 10 consecutive patients who are obese what risks they have of developing diabetes. Are their perspectives realistic?

Exercise 8

Having read through the material in this chapter, do you have a good understanding of the various complications of diabetes? Or do you need to read and study more? You could look up the original references cited in this chapter.

Now that you have completed these interactive reflection exercises, transfer the information to the relevant section about your learning needs in the empty template on pages 101–10 if you are working on your own personal development plan, or to the practice personal and professional development plan on pages 127–33 if you are working on a practice team learning plan. Don't forget to keep the evidence of your learning in your personal portfolio.

CHAPTER 5

Striving for optimal control

Intensive treatment of diabetes and hypertension reduces the development and progression of microvascular and neuropathic complications. The risk of development or progression of complications increases progressively as the glycosylated haemoglobin value increases above the non-diabetic range.[17]

Striving for normoglycaemia requires many restrictions to personal freedom. The frustration caused by these restrictions is illustrated in Box 5.1.

Box 5.1

One study demonstrated the perceived disadvantageous effects that diabetes has on the quality of life.[41] The researchers studied 292 patients whose age ranged from 21 to 85 years (mean age 62 years) and concluded that 'the average diabetic was willing to trade away 12% of his or her remaining life in return for a diabetic-free health state'.

There are two main aims of treatment for diabetes:

1 to allow as normal a daily life as possible without symptoms while at the same time avoiding acute complications such as ketoacidosis, hypoglycaemia and infection
2 to prevent or delay the long-term specific complications of diabetes, including microangiopathy (retinopathy, nephropathy), cataract and neuropathy, and to decrease the excess morbidity and mortality from macrovascular disease.[42]

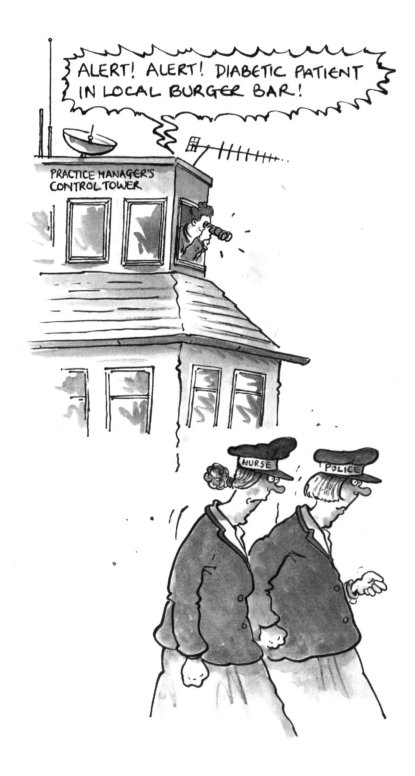

The benefits of control of type 1 diabetes mellitus

The better the glycaemic control, the more effective is primary and secondary prevention of retinal, renal and neurological complications.[5,14]

We have a great deal of evidence of the beneficial effects of improved blood glucose control in preventing and slowing the development of complications in diabetes. The risk of developing microvascular complications is substantially reduced if patients with type 1 diabetes achieve a glycosylated haemoglobin (HbA_{1c}) value of 7.5% or less, according to the Diabetes Control and Complications Trial described in Box 5.2.

Box 5.2 Summary of the Diabetes Control and Complications Trial (DCCT)[14]

- This randomised controlled trial was conducted in the USA from 1986.
- A total of 1441 patients with type 1 diabetes were randomly allocated to either 'intensive insulin therapy' (IIT) or conventional therapy.
- In total, 99% of diabetic subjects completed the study (except for those who died).
- The results showed that IIT delays the onset and slows the progression of diabetic retinopathy, nephropathy and neuropathy.
- Any improvement in the control of diabetes prevents complications – the better the control, the fewer the complications.
- IIT increased the risk of severe hypoglycaemia occurring by threefold.
- The results were so convincing that the trial was terminated after an average of 6.5 years.

The benefits of control of type 2 diabetes mellitus

The United Kingdom Prospective Diabetes Study (UKPDS)[15] showed that intensive control of blood glucose and tight control of blood pressure reduced the risk of microvascular complications. The findings of the study are summarised in Box 5.3. Tight glycaemic control was classified as glycosylated haemoglobin (HbA_{1c}) levels of 7.0% or less. Tight blood pressure control may be easier to achieve than tight glycaemic control for some individuals, and it has fewer side-effects and more of an impact on survival.

Any reduction in HbA_{1c} levels is likely to reduce the risk of complications, with the lowest risk being for HbA_{1c} values in the normal range – that is less than 6.0%. Each 1% reduction in mean HbA_{1c} levels was associated with a 21% reduction in deaths related to diabetes.[43]

Box 5.3 Summary of the United Kingdom Prospective Diabetes Study (UKPDS)[5,15]

- The UKPDS was a multicentre randomised controlled trial conducted in the UK from 1977.
- A total of 4209 patients aged 25–65 years with newly diagnosed type 2 diabetes were randomly allocated to different therapies, namely 'conventional' diet and exercise therapy, or 'intensive' diet and exercise *and* oral hypoglycaemic or insulin therapy.
- Over the 10 years of the study, the mean HbA_{1c} value in the intensively treated group was lower than that in the conventionally treated group (7.0% vs. 7.9% HbA_{1c}).
- The risk for any diabetes-related end-point in the 'intensive' group was 12% lower than that in the 'conventional' group.
- The absolute risk of death was 46 deaths per 1000 patient years in the 'intensive' group compared to 41 deaths per 1000 patient years in the 'conventional' group. This difference in glycaemic control was not statistically significant.
- There was a 25% reduction in the risk of the microvascular end-points between the two groups, from 11.4 events to 8.6 events per 1000 patient years.
- There was no significant difference in any of the diabetes-related end-points between therapy with chlorpropamide, glibenclamide or insulin.
- The lower mean blood pressure in the tight blood pressure control group of 144/82 mmHg compared with 154/87 mmHg was translated into lower risks of serious complications, namely 32% less deaths, 44% less strokes and 37% less microvascular end-point damage.
- Most of the subjects who were randomised to the blood pressure control groups needed more than one antihypertensive treatment to control their blood pressure effectively.

Modifying risk factors

Smoking

Smoking is associated with poor glycaemic control. Microvascular complications are more common and progress more quickly.

Box 5.4

A study in Atlanta, USA, showed that people with diabetes are as likely to smoke as those without diabetes. More than 40% of smokers with diabetes reported that their doctor had not advised or helped them to stop smoking.[5]

Obesity

If we could influence obese people in the general population to reduce their weight and sustain it at a lower level, then far fewer people would develop type 2 diabetes. Unfortunately, however, the proportion of people with obesity in the general population continues to rise despite greater awareness of obesity as a potential problem, and a plethora of local health promotion activities.

Three out of four people with newly diagnosed type 2 diabetes are obese – that is, their body mass index is 30 or more. Obesity worsens insulin resistance.

Box 5.5

An American study that followed people with impaired glucose tolerance (the state between diabetes and normal glucose metabolism) over four years found that if they improved their diet and increased their exercise levels, they more than halved the rate at which diabetes was newly diagnosed. This was achieved by seven, hour-long meetings with a dietitian in the first year and quarterly thereafter, and opportunities for supervised exercise three times a week.[44]

Weight loss not only lowers blood glucose, but also lowers lipid levels and blood pressure, all of which are significant risk factors for type 2 diabetes. In addition, smoking cessation, reducing excessive alcohol intake and regular physical activity all reduce the risk of macrovascular complications occurring.

Diet

Lipid lowering

People with all types of diabetes need full lipid profiles determined annually rather than random cholesterol tests. If the lipid profile remains abnormal after initial treatment, they should be re-tested after three months. The UKPDS trial demonstrated the association between raised lipids and death rates (from cardiovascular disease, heart attack, stroke, peripheral vascular disease, hypo- and hyperglycaemia and sudden deaths). Every reduction of 1 mmol/L in total cholesterol was associated with a 24% reduction in diabetes-related deaths over the 10.4-year average follow-up period of the study. A 1 mmol/L decrease in LDL-cholesterol reduced diabetes-related deaths by 25% and a 0.1 mmol/L increase in HDL-cholesterol was associated with a 7% reduction in diabetes-related deaths.[15]

High fibre

A high-fibre diet reduced blood glucose levels in 13 patients with type 2 diabetes in another study, a similar reduction to that achieved by the addition of an oral hypoglycaemic drug. Plasma glucose, plasma cholesterol, triglyceride and plasma insulin levels were all lower when patients were on a 50 g/day high-fibre diet compared to one with a moderate fibre intake of 24 g/day.[45]

Eating disorders

Box 5.6

A Canadian study of adolescent diabetic girls has shown that eating disorders are two to three times more common in young diabetic females than in age-matched controls.[46] This is particularly important as mean HbA_{1c} levels were higher in those with eating disorders, putting them at increased risk of complications.

Preventing complications

Preventing renal complications[18,23]

The urine of patients with type 2 diabetes should be tested at least annually for proteinuria and, if negative, for microalbuminuria.

In patients with microalbuminuria or proteinuria, treatment with angiotensin-converting enzyme (ACE) inhibitors is appropriate even if blood pressure is normal. People with type 1 diabetes who have confirmed microalbuminuria should be referred to a specialist clinic for investigation.

Blood glucose levels should be kept as near to normal as is consistent with an acceptable quality of life.

Blood pressure should be checked regularly and treatment offered or changed if one reading of either the systolic pressure is >140 mmHg or the diastolic pressure is > 80 mmHg.

Preventing complications from foot disease

Tight control of blood glucose and blood pressure is the key. Risk factors such as smoking and raised lipid levels should be minimised. In addition, current guidelines recommend the following.[19,47]

- Patients with diabetes who have no clinical evidence of neuro-pathy or peripheral vascular disease require general foot education and regular risk assessment at an annual review. The annual screening examination of the feet should include assessment of peripheral neuropathy, peripheral circulation, skin condition and deformity.
- Patients who are 'at risk' include those with previous foot ulceration (an extremely high-risk group), neuropathy, peripheral vascular disease, callus, foot deformity, partial sight, physical disability, the elderly and those who are living alone. These patients should have regular intensive foot care education and chiropody follow-up, either at a specialist diabetic chiropody clinic in the community or at a hospital diabetic foot clinic. Their feet should be inspected every 3–6 months and they should be referred if they need a vascular assessment.
- Patients with 'high-risk' feet require frequent review by a podiatrist or foot care team every 1–3 months, to evaluate whether intense foot

care education, specialist footwear and insoles, and skin and nail care is appropriate. Review the need for vascular assessment, and take special care of those with disabilities or immobility.

Box 5.7

An annual foot screen for everyone with any type of diabetes should include inspection of the feet, including palpation of pulses and testing of sensitivity to fine touch, to identify those people with 'at risk' feet.

Future developments

A possible future treatment option for diabetes is that of islet-cell transplantation.[48] This procedure is minimally invasive compared with transplantation of the whole pancreas, but studies so far have found that only 8% of recipients were still insulin independent one year after the operation.

Transplantation of a whole pancreas has been performed on 15 000 patients. One year on, 85% of the grafts had survived and recipients were still producing enough insulin for their needs. Such pancreatic transplants may prevent and ameliorate the progression of complications from diabetes. However, the improved quality of life may not justify the combined risks of immunosuppression and major surgery.

Simultaneous pancreas–kidney transplantation is the treatment of choice for patients with diabetes and end-stage renal disease.

Targets for metabolic control and the control of cardiovascular risk factors in people with diabetes

As more research is published, existing guidelines become outdated and the goals of treatment become tighter and more challenging. Box 5.8 shows the consensus that seems to be emerging from the various guidelines, presented here as a spectrum of good to poor control for the most important risk factors.

Box 5.8 Targets for metabolic control and the control of cardiovascular risk factors in people with diabetes[15,17,38,49]

	Good	Borderline	Poor
Total cholesterol (mmol/L)	< 5.0	5.0–6.5	> 6.5
HDL-cholesterol (mmol/L)	> 1.1	0.9–1.1	< 0.9
Fasting triglycerides (mmol/L)	< 1.7	1.7–2.2	> 2.2
Body mass index (kg/m^2)			
Males	20–25	26–27	> 27
Females	19–24	25–26	> 26
Blood pressure (mmHg)	< 130/80*	140/80**–160/95	> 160/95
Smoking status	Non-smoker	Smoker	Smoker

* Varies according to different guidelines. Stricter targets are advocated for younger people and for individuals with microvascular or macrovascular complications.
** UKPDS recommends that treatment is indicated if above 140/80.

Managing the risks of coronary heart disease and raised lipids

Treating people with statins reduces the risk of myocardial infarction by about 30% and the risk of death by about 20–30% over five years, regardless of the baseline risk of cardiovascular disease. The benefits are similar whether or not people have diabetes. This is the basis of the argument for putting patients with type 2 diabetes on statins if they have normal cholesterol levels but abnormal triglyceride or HDL values. Experts argue that it is not appropriate, for those with diabetes, to base treatment decisions about using lipid-lowering drugs on the presence of individual cardiovascular risk factors viewed in isolation. Treatment should be instituted if the overall risk of myocardial infarction is assessed as being 30% or higher over 10 years.

Similarly good results in terms of reductions in cardiovascular risk have been found for people with diabetes treated with fibrates, with a

22% reduction in the risk of vascular events being reported in one major trial.[17] Several large trials are evaluating the effects of fibrates in people with diabetes.

Use appropriate tables to assess the risk of cardiovascular disease before deciding when to use lipid-lowering treatment (or other treatments) in the primary prevention of cardiovascular disease.[17,49,50] A copy of a suitable risk table can be found at the back of an up-to-date *British National Formulary*[51] or other compendium.[38] As a general guide, an absolute risk of 15% or higher of developing cardiovascular disease over the next 10 years is sufficient to justify lipid-lowering drug treatment in primary prevention in diabetic patients.[49,51] Statin doses should be adequate in order to reduce total cholesterol to recommended levels.

Diabetes is such a significant risk factor for coronary heart disease that, when using the risk assessment guidelines,[49,51] the primary prevention of coronary heart disease in patients with diabetes approximates to the secondary prevention of coronary heart disease in people with normal glucose tolerance.

Management of hypertension in people with diabetes

Around 40% of people with type 2 diabetes have a raised blood pressure and are therefore at risk of developing myocardial infarction and premature death.[52] Tight control of blood pressure to below 130/80 mmHg may be a more effective method of preventing diabetic complications in people with diabetes who have a systolic blood pressure of >159 mmHg than tight control of blood glucose (fasting level below 6 mmol/L).[49] The number of patients who develop any diabetes-related end-point is six for tight blood pressure control compared with 20 for tight blood glucose control.[52] Any reduction in blood pressure is likely to reduce the risk of complications, with the lowest risk being found in individuals with systolic blood pressures of less than 120 mmHg.[53]

The reduction in blood pressure seems to matter more than the particular drug used. Many patients with type 2 diabetes need a combination of antihypertensive agents to maintain low blood pressure.[52] Around one-third of the subjects who were included in the UKPDS trial required three or more antihypertensive treatments to achieve effective blood pressure control.[49,54]

Type 2 diabetes is more than twice as likely to occur in people with hypertension as in people with normal blood pressure. In one major study it was found that diabetes was more common in individuals with hypertension taking beta-blocker drugs than in those receiving no treatment, whereas patients taking thiazides were slightly less likely to develop diabetes.[55] Calcium-channel blockers and ACE inhibitors represented no greater risk to developing diabetes than was found in those not receiving such antihypertensive treatment. The conclusion of the study was that 'concern about the risk of diabetes should not discourage doctors from prescribing thiazide diuretics to non-diabetic adults who have hypertension', and that beta-blocker drugs should continue to be prescribed. The adverse effect of increasing the risk of diabetes must be weighed against the proven benefits of controlling hypertension and reducing the risk of cardiovascular events.

The ACE inhibitor ramipril lowered the risk of myocardial infarction, stroke and cardiovascular death when it was taken by patients with diabetes with at least one other cardiovascular risk factor.[56] The conclusion was that the risk reduction could not simply be attributed to the drug's antihypertensive effect.

Management of blood glucose

The treatment cascade

Diet is the first line of treatment for people with type 2 diabetes. Try diet for three months. People who are overweight should try to lose weight by both restricting the energy and carbohydrate content of their diet and increasing their physical activity. Add a sulphonylurea or metformin if the diet and exercise are not successful in controlling blood glucose. Increase the dose of tablets as appropriate, and add a second oral drug if necessary – the usual combination is a sulphonylurea with metformin or acarbose. If diabetes is still insufficiently controlled, switch to a combination of insulin and oral medication, or insulin therapy alone.[57]

Oral hypoglycaemic agents

Sulphonylureas and insulin have a good safety profile. They do not increase the cardiovascular risk. Metformin is a good first-line therapy in overweight patients with type 2 diabetes, if there are no contraindications.[58]

Box 5.9 Poor adherence to oral hypoglycaemic therapy[59]

Two-thirds of patients with type 2 diabetes did not adhere to their prescribed oral hypoglycaemic treatment in a study undertaken in Scotland. Only 31% of patients who were prescribed sulphonyl-ureas alone and 34% of those who were prescribed metformin alone adhered to their medication, which was taken for an average of 300 out of 365 days per year. Patients on combination treatment with a sulphonylurea plus metformin showed dramatically poorer compliance, with only 13% adhering to their medication regime, which was taken on an average of 266 out of 365 days per year.

People who were most likely to adhere to their recommended treatment were:

- on monotherapy
- those with diabetes of shorter duration
- on fewer co-medications
- less socially deprived individuals.

Sulphonlyureas (e.g. glibenclamide, gliclazide, glimepiride, glipizide)

Sulphonylureas are the first-line treatment in normal-weight patients with type 2 diabetes. They act by stimulating secretion of insulin from functioning pancreatic beta-cells. Sulphonylurea therapy satisfactorily controls glycaemia in about two-thirds of patients with type 2 diabetes. Hyperinsulinaemia can occur, and may lead to hypoglycaemia and weight gain. If hypoglycaemia occurs, the dose should be reduced.

Biguanides (e.g. metformin)

Metformin is a first-line treatment for people with type 2 diabetes who are overweight. Biguanides lower blood glucose levels by inhibiting hepatic glucose production. Adverse effects are common and include gastrointestinal symptoms, and (rarely) lactic acidosis. Avoid using metformin in patients with heart failure, or with kidney or liver failure.

Alpha-glucosidase inhibitors (e.g. acarbose)

These drugs delay glucose absorption from the intestine, thus reducing post-prandial glucose levels, and they are an add-on treatment. They may cause flatulence, diarrhoea or abdominal bloating, so should be avoided in individuals with irritable bowel syndrome.

Prandial glucose regulators (e.g. repaglinide)

These drugs are short-acting oral secretagogues, lowering blood glucose levels by the stimulation of insulin release from the pancreas. This action clearly depends on functioning beta-cells in the pancreatic islets.

Glitazones (e.g. rosiglitazone, pioglitazone)

These relatively new drugs act on the nuclear receptors in adipose tissue, which are termed the perixisome proliferator-activated receptors. Glitazones target the gamma receptors to influence lipid and glucose metabolism, glucose transport and storage. They also reduce atherogenesis by direct effects on the vascular wall and coagulation.
Glitazones can postpone insulin therapy for those with type 2 diabetes by preventing the decline in pancreatic beta-cell function and preserving endogenous insulin secretion.

The side-effects of glitazones include weight gain (about 3 kg over six months), ankle swelling (which is unrelated to heart failure) and a slight reduction in haemoglobin.

The National Institute for Clinical Excellence (NICE) has approved rosiglitazone for use in England. It is effective in reducing blood glucose levels when added to oral monotherapy (metformin or sulphonylurea) for patients who have inadequate control of blood glucose on these conventional drugs alone. If control is inadequate on oral monotherapy, the patient should be offered combination therapy with metformin and sulphonylurea, so long as the combination is tolerated. If patients cannot tolerate the combination therapy or their blood glucose level remains high, then consider rosiglitazone in combination with metformin as an alternative to injected insulin. Use sulphonylurea in place of metformin if the latter is contraindicated or not tolerated. Liver function tests should be performed before therapy is initiated (two-monthly in the first year, with periodic checks thereafter). Rosiglitazone is contraindicated in patients with a history of cardiac failure, hepatic impairment or severe renal insufficiency.[60]

Insulin should be considered for type 2 patients who are not adequately controlled by diet and/or oral hypoglycaemic agents alone or in combination. Insulin can be used in combination therapy with oral hypoglycaemic drugs such as sulphonylureas and biguanides.

Box 5.10 Benefits of insulin treatment in type 2 diabetes[61]

A significant proportion of patients with type 2 diabetes require insulin treatment. A study of the benefits and adverse effects of insulin conversion in 236 diabetic subjects found that the majority of patients with type 2 diabetes who were poorly controlled by oral hypoglycaemics will benefit from the addition of insulin, if the HbA_{1c} value is above 9% at conversion. The strongest predictor of benefit was the initial HbA_{1c} value, but initial weight was also important. Better glycaemic control was gained at the expense of a significant weight gain and a significant rate of hypoglycaemia.

Sulphonylureas and insulin, but not metformin, increase the risks of weight gain and hypoglycaemia. In one report, the proportions of people per year with severe hypoglycaemic episodes were 1.2% for chlorpropamide, 1% for glibenclamide, 2% for insulin and 0.6% for metformin. There is no evidence that any specific hypoglycaemic agent increases the overall risk of cardiovascular disease.[17] Chlorpropamide and glibenclamide should be avoided in the elderly because of the greater risk of hypoglycaemia, and gliclazide or tolbutamide should be used instead.

Insulins

Insulin-dependent (type 1) or insulin-treated (type 2) patients need to be kept well informed and updated about why insulin is used, what type of insulin to use, how it is used (the technique) and when it is given. Patients should be alerted to the fact that the risk of hypoglycaemia is increased with tighter control of blood glucose.

Suggestions that human insulin reduces the early warning signs of a 'hypo' have not been supported by research evidence.

Usually the decision to introduce insulin has been negotiated with people with type 2 diabetes over a considerable period of time. The patient should understand the reasons why their blood glucose control is worse, and the advantages and drawbacks of insulin. They will probably have contributed to their management by self-monitoring of blood sugars. This phase of diabetes care can be very demanding, and it often requires the help of experts from outside the practice, depending on the capability of the practice nurse and the GP.

Patients should be taught the basic injection technique, the rotation of injection sites, and information about mixing insulins in the syringe – soluble (clear) with a longer acting (cloudy) insulin.

Timing of insulin

Sometimes patients can be managed on once-a-day intermediate-acting insulin or a mixture of short- and medium-acting insulin. This may be useful for someone with type 2 diabetes to add to oral hypoglycaemic agents, particularly for elderly patients, for whom twice daily injections may not be feasible.

A twice-a-day short- and medium-acting mixture is popular. The ratio of short- and medium-acting insulin can be varied to suit lifestyle, work and also residual endogenous insulin production. These will vary over time and need frequent reappraisal. Fixed mixtures of soluble and isophane insulins are available in a range of proportions.

A 'bolus' regime has been developed to give patients more flexibility. A short-acting insulin is given before each meal, and an intermediate-acting insulin is given before bedtime. Staying in balance requires considerable knowledge of diabetes by the patient and the practice nurse.

Pens are popular because they are portable and simple to use. There is also a version which is suitable for the visually impaired. There is an upper limit of 76 units in the insulin cartridges.

Management of peripheral neuropathy

The pain of peripheral neuropathy is best managed by aiming for steady levels of blood glucose and avoiding swings, rather than by instituting any particular treatment. Only the maintenance of near normo-glycaemia slows down the progress of the neuropathy. There is no evidence that any symptomatic treatments influence the natural history of neuropathy. Tricyclic drugs are commonly used as first-line agents to control severe pain, although they are not licensed for this treatment. Some authors advocate the use of carbamazepine and gabapentin for controlling neuropathic pain, but the relative efficacy of these drugs has not been determined.[62]

Management of microalbuminuria

ACE inhibitors reduce albumin excretion in people with diabetes with microalbuminuria and normal blood pressure.[63] ACE inhibitors can be prescribed to all patients with type 2 diabetes with raised levels of protein in their urine, whether or not they have hypertension.[23] Practically, this means that every patient with type 2 diabetes should have an annual renal function check for proteinuria and, if this is negative, a check for microalbuminuria. *See* Figure 7.1.

Management of foot problems

The main recommendations for managing foot care for all people with diabetes[47] are as follows:

1 to undertake an annual review of complications and risk factors with trained personnel (*see* Chapter 7 on the practice-based approach)
2 to classify foot risk as
   • 'low current risk' – normal sensation, palpable pulses
   • 'at risk' – neuropathy or absent pulses or other risk factor(s)
   • 'high risk' – risk factor and deformity or skin change or previous ulcer
   • 'ulcerated foot'.

Tight blood glucose and blood pressure control are important when managing patients with foot problems, just as described in the section on prevention of foot problems earlier in this chapter. Management of a foot ulcer should include referral for an expert opinion, investigation and treatment of vascular insufficiency, good local wound management, systemic antibiotic therapy for cellulitis or bone infection, effective footwear and aids for distributing pressure points across the foot. Spreading cellulitis (a hot foot) should be treated as a medical emergency and seen urgently by the specialist service in secondary care.

Management of hypoglycaemic episodes

The emphasis on tighter blood glucose control and lower levels of blood glucose may trigger more frequent episodes of hypoglycaemia – for those taking oral hypoglycaemic drugs as well as those on insulin. People with diabetes should carry dextrose or some other form of carbohydrate with them at all times to take when they experience the warning signs of hypoglycaemia, such as tremor, sweating, confusion, irritability, racing pulse or poor co-ordination. Carers or parents should be educated to watch out for signs of a hypoglycaemic attack (hypo) and intercede if the patient does not take action. A parent or carer can administer one unit of glucagon subcutaneously or intramuscularly to treat a hypo if the dextrose or other carbohydrate has not worked. An intravenous load of 50% glucose must be given by a clinician 10 minutes later if there is no response to the glucagon. People with diabetes should be encouraged to carry a card or bracelet describing their diagnosis and the treatment that they take.

Reflection exercises

Exercise 9

Review the extent to which you are successful in helping patients with diabetes to gain optimal control over their blood glucose and blood pressure, and to minimise complications.

Randomly select 20 case notes from patients with type 1 diabetes, and a further random selection of 20 case notes of those with type 2 diabetes (controlled by oral therapy and insulin or diet), and compare how well controlled their various risk factors are against the goals you are aiming for:[17,38]

1 blood pressure
2 HbA$_{1c}$
3 smoking status
4 lipid levels – total cholesterol, HDL-cholesterol, fasting triglycerides
5 body mass index.

What do you and your team need to learn from this exercise, and what reorganisation of the practice do you need to arrange? Repeat the exercise for the high-risk group of patients with diabetes and coronary heart disease.

Exercise 10

Identify those patients in the practice who have had previous foot ulcers. For this high-risk group, check that:

1 they are receiving ongoing care from a podiatrist
2 the glycaemic control is optimal.

Now that you have completed this interactive reflection exercise, transfer the information to the relevant section about your learning needs in the empty template on pages 101–10 if you are working on your own personal development plan, or to the practice personal and professional development plan on pages 127–33 if you are working on a practice team learning plan. Don't forget to keep the evidence of your learning in your personal portfolio.

CHAPTER 6

Patient-centred care

People with diabetes[34] should:

- be aware of the importance of maintaining good control of their diabetes
- try to lose weight if they are overweight or obese
- eat a low-fat, high-fibre diet
- stop smoking
- take exercise.

Self-monitoring

Published studies provide conflicting results about the usefulness of self-monitoring of blood glucose levels. Some still advocate self-monitoring of glucose control, but a recent report from the Health Technology Assessment (HTA)[64] programme has indicated that self-monitoring in type 2 diabetes may be unnecessary. The HTA found that regular self-testing is uncommon even in patients with type 1 diabetes. There was no evidence to show that self-monitoring of blood or urine glucose by individuals with type 2 diabetes improves blood glucose control measured by HbA_{1c} or fasting plasma glucose, nor was blood glucose monitoring more effective than urine glucose monitoring. However, some of the studies that were reviewed were poorly conducted and reported so that small but clinically relevant effects might not have been detectable.

Patients with type 1 diabetes who regularly self-monitored were better controlled, but this may have reflected a greater level of adherence to other aspects of diabetes self-management. The HTA report urges that people with type 1 diabetes or unstable type 2 diabetes should be monitored by clinicians measuring their HbA_{1c} four times per year.

Patients with diabetes should be more aware of the importance of HbA_{1c} in the monitoring of their condition and view self-monitoring of blood glucose levels as an adjunct to overall monitoring. Unless the findings of the HTA report are clearly explained to patients, those who have conscientiously carried out regular self-monitoring of blood glucose will be bewildered. However, for patients with type 2 diabetes who prefer urine testing to blood glucose monitoring, the HTA report is good news.

Urine testing for glucose is of less value than blood glucose testing because urine glucose concentration does not vary directly with blood glucose levels. The urine should be tested for ketones when blood or urine glucose levels are high. Ketones indicate a severe level of metabolic disturbance that needs corrective treatment to reduce the hyperglycaemia.

Patient education leading to patient empowerment

The importance of good patient education was emphasised in the conclusions of a systematic review: 'The key to care lies first in patient education: the patient needs to know and understand the full situation about his or her disease and to be empowered to receive the maximum amount of care possible in their own home and within their own family . . . The disease is frightening, restricting and irritating . . .' 'What has to be achieved is a working partnership between patient and (health) carers'. 'Empowerment should be a central goal for both patients and professionals'.[65]

The study illustrated in Box 6.1 below describes one team's efforts to rate the quality of patient education. You might adapt it for your own requirements.

Box 6.1 A diabetes knowledge assessment tool to improve provision of patient education[66]

A knowledge assessment tool based on assessment of a patient's ability to manage diabetes was developed in-house for use by the diabetes team in Bolton. The extent of knowledge is scored as follows:

1   patient has no knowledge of issue
2   patient has non-functional knowledge of issue

3 patient has basic functional knowledge of issue
4 patient is fully conversant with most aspects of issue.

The scores are applied to each item on a 'check-list' of highly important factors in the patient's disease management (e.g. ability to understand treatment, manage hypoglycaemia and foot care). For each item in the check-list a comprehensive set of guidelines exists to ensure that staff teach patients about all of the key components. This type of scoring system will facilitate decision making and help to shape education to meet individual patient needs. It will also provide auditable standards.

The St Vincent Declaration stated that improving health and preventing complications in people with diabetes will only be achieved with the active participation of such individuals through patient empowerment.[67] A recent survey substantiated this (see Box 6.2).

Box 6.2 Do people with diabetes desire a role in diabetes treatment decision?[68]

Most of the 450 respondents to a recent postal survey in the UK felt confident that they were capable of making choices about their treatment (91% vs. 78% for insulin and oral medication users, respectively). In total, 46% of insulin-only patients and <15% of orally treated patients felt that they knew more about controlling their diabetes than their professional caregivers did. Most diabetic patients wanted to discuss and be involved in treatment decisions, but still regarded healthcare professionals, rather than themselves, as the ultimate diabetes experts.

The Diabetes UK 'Patients' Charter'[69] emphasises a patient's right to good information throughout their management and care, and their right to be involved in decision making about their management. A registered nurse with a special interest in diabetes should explain what diabetes is and talk to the patient about their individual treatment. A state-registered dietitian should give the patient basic advice on what to eat in the future. Discussion with the patient should cover the implications of diabetes for their job, driving, insurance, prescription charges, etc., as well as ongoing education about their diabetes and its control and the beneficial effects of exercise.

For patients on insulin there should be frequent instruction on injection technique, looking after their insulin and syringes, blood glucose and ketone testing and what the results mean, and when, why and how to deal with hypoglycaemia. For those on oral therapy, there should be a discussion about the possibility of hypoglycaemic attacks ('hypos') and how to deal with them, instruction on blood or urine testing and explanation of the results. For those being managed by diet alone, an explanation of the potential risks from obesity and coexisting cardiovascular disease should be given, together with instruction on blood or urine testing and explanation of results.

Box 6.3

Diabetes UK emphasises that the person with diabetes is an important member of the care team, and therefore it is essential that they understand about diabetes to enable them to be in control of their own diabetic condition.

The importance of patient education is shown in the study described in Box 6.4. Integrated care pathways map expected care, improve implementation of guidelines, facilitate critical evaluation of care and improve communication within multidisciplinary teams. In this study, integrated care pathway-driven diabetes education was associated with highly significant improvements.

Box 6.4 Diabetes education is associated with improvements in diabetes knowledge, diabetes well-being and HbA_{1c}[70]

One prospective study of the impact of a formal integrated care pathway-driven education programme on HbA_{1c} compared patients' knowledge and well-being at weeks 0 and 6, and HbA_{1c} at weeks 0 and 12. There were highly significant improvements in diabetes knowledge, diabetes well-being and HbA_{1c} (8.7 to 7.6, $P < 0.0001$) compared to the baseline.

A study of 261 patients with type 2 diabetes attending two diabetes centres revealed a great deal of ignorance about their medication, including how it worked and possible side-effects. Only 15% of the subjects knew how their medication worked and 62% took their tablets correctly in relation to food. Only 10% of those who were taking a sulphonylurea knew that it might cause hypoglycaemia, and only 20%

of those taking metformin were aware of its gastrointestinal side-effects. About 20% forgot to take their medication at least once a week and 5% mistakenly omitted tablets, misunderstanding the dose. A parallel study of health professionals' knowledge also showed gaps in their knowledge about dosage timing and the mechanism of action of the oral hypoglycaemic drugs (e.g. that sulphonylurea drugs should be taken with or before breakfast, depending on the exact drug, whereas metformin is taken in divided doses).[71]

Box 6.5 Cardiovascular risk perception in patients with type 2 diabetes[72]

Research investigating the beliefs of patients with type 2 diabetes with regard to cardiovascular risk found that most patients had a basic understanding of the concept of cardiovascular risk, but rated their own risk in accordance with their personal beliefs. Although most of them had some knowledge of medical risk factors, few associated being diabetic with increased risk. Patients who wished to preserve their perceived quality of life rather than adopt the lifestyle advocated by health professionals justified their choice with personal health beliefs and anecdotal evidence. Patients' perceptions of risk differed significantly from those of physicians, in that they relied more on personal experience and health beliefs, whereas clinicians used clinical measures and judgement. This reduced patients' compliance with risk-reducing behaviour and medication, and it has implications for improving patient education.

The better the patient's relationship with the treating doctor or nurse, and the more opportunity there is for discussion, the more likely it is that their fears or mistaken beliefs about treatment can be expressed and defused or corrected.

One recent study has cautioned against too intense a patient-centred relationship, suggesting that this diverts attention from the more clinical aspects of diabetes management. When patients who had been looked after by doctors and nurses who had received training in adopting a patient-centred approach were compared with patients who had been looked after by those who had not received such training, there was no significant difference in glycaemic control. However, those in the group that received more care from the doctors and nurses who had been trained in being patient-centred had higher body mass indices and triglyceride levels, and less knowledge about their disease.[73]

The child's view

Children and adolescents need help to limit the effects of diabetes on school life and their career goals. The primary care team is best placed to persuade adolescents not to default from clinic visits and to maintain clinical contact through to adulthood. The guidelines[74] recommend that:

- all children with diabetes are cared for by a multidisciplinary hospital-based team including a paediatrician, a paediatric specialist nurse and a dietitian with special expertise in childhood diabetes
- all those in the general practice team caring for young diabetic patients have well-defined roles
- there is good liaison between primary care services and schools
- special problems faced by teenagers with diabetes should be recognised and contact systems developed for defaulters
- audit and research are well co-ordinated around local registers of diabetic patients.

Box 6.6 What is it like to be a child with diabetes?[75]

One GP who has had diabetes since childhood offers the following advice.

- Encourage parents to stay with their child in hospital.
- Children with diabetes become adept at manipulating adults' fears.
- Children do remember unpleasant medical procedures – so help them to adjust to the memories.
- Children are entitled to privacy in the same way as adults are.
- Parents should try to treat a child with diabetes as normally as possible in order to minimise the impact of the chronic disease on his or her life.

Improving compliance and concordance[76]

Encourage patients to comply with a sensible lifestyle, treatment and self-care by using a SMART approach. That is, agree **S**pecific objectives with them that are **M**easurable with targets that are **A**chievable, **R**elevant and **T**ime-specific. People should know what they are aiming for and whether they have attained those goals.

Give patients with diabetes a full explanation of diabetes and the potential complications of the condition soon after they have been diagnosed. Many of those with type 2 diabetes mistakenly believe that their condition is not serious because they have had an inadequate explanation of the facts. They may have a false sense of security while they are in the asymptomatic phase. They need to understand the importance of tightening blood glucose and blood pressure control as an investment in their future health and well-being. Use simple language, and avoid swamping patients with complicated statistics if they are not ready for them or cannot understand such detailed information.

Patients with diabetes comply most closely with their prescribed medication if it can be taken once a day. A study of the extent to which people with type 2 diabetes comply with their treatment found that less than one-third of those who were prescribed one oral hypoglycaemic drug took their medication for 90% or more of the time. If more than one hypoglycaemic drug was prescribed, or additional drugs were prescribed for other conditions, only one-sixth took their medication on most days.

Why don't patients comply with their treatment?[77] Reasons for this include the following:

- lack of education or understanding about the importance of daily treatment
- confusion about which tablets to take and when, especially in the elderly or those with learning difficulties
- changes in drug or dosage regimens
- unpleasant side-effects
- physical difficulties in opening the packaging or problems with reading the labels
- the demands of a busy lifestyle.

Consider how to motivate patients to adhere to their prescribed medication and a sensible lifestyle. Understanding their values, beliefs and preferences, and whether they are optimists or pessimists by nature, will enable you to tailor the style and content of your health messages to the individual patient.

Box 6.7

The demands of a busy lifestyle can make it difficult for a person with diabetes to comply with regular treatment and monitoring.[78]

> 'As a newly diagnosed person with type 2 diabetes myself, I now realise that even taking one tablet daily, in addition to other aspects of self-care and regular visits to my GP's practice, takes time in my already hectic life.'
>
> People with type 2 diabetes who work irregular shifts find it really difficult to keep good glycaemic control without running the risk of hypoglycaemic attacks that might endanger themselves or their colleagues at work.

Diabetes UK reports that only 20% of people aged over 50 years who have diabetes are in employment compared to one-third of those without diabetes of the same age group.[34]

Reflection exercises

Exercise 11

Locate all the patient literature you have in your practice for people with diabetes. Does the literature match the most up-to-date thinking about best practice in diabetes management? Or does it promote out-of-date practices and approaches, or use old terminology such as 'non-insulin-dependent' instead of 'type 2'? You need to be clear yourself about the most up-to-date recommendations in order to be able to check your literature and complete this exercise.

Exercise 12

Find out what initiatives have been undertaken by any members of the practice team in order to ascertain patients' views in the previous 12 months. This might have included surveying or involving anyone registered with the practice (e.g. regular patients, people who do not use the services, carers) or the local community. How was the information gathered from the initiative used? Did changes occur as a result? Your own or practice team members' learning needs from this exercise might include the following:

- learning more about the variety of methods that can be employed to ascertain patients' views
- learning how to apply any of those methods to ascertain the views of

people with diabetes about the care or services that are provided or that they wish to receive
- learning more about organising a survey so that the findings are useful for making changes to the way in which services are planned or delivered, or the way in which staff behave
- learning more about involving individual patients in decision making about the management of their diabetes.

Now that you have completed these interactive reflection exercises, transfer the information to the relevant section about your learning needs in the empty template on pages 101–10 if you are working on your own personal development plan, or to the practice personal and professional development plan on pages 127–33 if you are working on a practice team learning plan. Don't forget to keep the evidence of your learning in your personal portfolio.

CHAPTER 7

A practice-based approach to providing good diabetic care

The St Vincent Declaration of 1989[67] sets out important goals for the care of those with diabetes which should be central to your practice protocol. These goals are listed in Box 7.1.

Box 7.1 St Vincent targets for those with diabetes (in brief)[67]

- To decrease retinopathic blindness and renal failure by one-third or more.
- To halve amputations due to diabetic gangrene.
- To reduce morbidity and mortality from cardiovascular disease and stroke.
- To normalise the outcome of pregnancy.

To meet the St Vincent goals, the aims of diabetes care should include:[5]

- opportunistic screening of those at high risk of diabetes
- involvement of all those identified in a planned programme of care
- ensuring that all those with diabetes and their carers have access to appropriate education
- maintaining optimal metabolic control to prevent or delay the development of complications
- eliminating the acute problems of hypo- and hyperglycaemia
- ensuring the early identification and treatment of complications
- improving glycaemic control in pregnancy.

Compiling or updating a diabetic register

Most practices have a diabetic register, but yours may not be as up to date as it should be. You could use the check-list below every so often to see that your register includes the details of all the patients with diabetes.

- Record or check the names of patients with diabetes as you encounter them in surgery or on visits, and ensure that they are included on the register.
- Search the repeat-prescription system for patients receiving prescriptions for insulin, oral hypoglycaemics, insulin syringes or urine- or blood-testing reagents.
- Ask the district nurses, community pharmacists, optometrists and other members of the team to recall diabetic patients' identities.
- Ask the local optometrist or hospital-based diabetic clinics for the names of your patients attending.

Make sure that the diagnosis is coded on the practice computer using Read codes from the national minimum dataset. The commonest mistake is for older people requiring insulin to be coded as type 1 instead of type 2.

Primary care, shared care or hospital-based care?

There seems to be a consensus on recommendations for standards of diabetic care.[65]

- All people with diabetes should be receiving preventative care from a diabetes team with education and medical interventions aimed at normalising metabolic state according to published targets while at the same time maintaining quality of life.
- All people with diabetes should have immediate and continuing access to a diabetes team (in primary or secondary care) in order to deal with changes in metabolic state, concerns about diabetes, and social difficulties arising from their condition.
- All people with diabetes should have access to an annual review for complications of diabetes, and that where a failure of preventative care is detected a suitable care plan should be made to manage the complication, and such a plan must be adequately implemented.
- People with diabetes have a major role to play not only in their

self-management, but also in the development of the service of which they are a part.

Diabetes teams should be examining the success of care delivered at least annually, through aggregation of the results of metabolic outcome measures and true adverse patient outcomes.

People with diabetes in any locality should be recorded on a register, which should be updated annually to confirm that the activities described above actually occurred. Appropriate special care is offered to some groups of people with diabetes and special needs, such as pregnant women.

The results of a meta-analysis by the Cochrane Diabetes Group of five trials suggest that 'prompted' primary care which includes a system of recall and regular review of diabetes can be as effective as hospital care in terms of glycaemic control. Such prompted care is better than hospital care in terms of maintaining contact with patients.[5] The effective element appears to be the computerised recall with prompting for patients and their family doctors. The extent to which care should be 'shared' between the hospital team and primary care is likely to vary from one practice to another, from patient to patient and from time to time for any one patient when there are problems or they are vulnerable to complications.

Box 7.2 Proportion of diabetic care taking place in the community[79]

A survey of diabetes care in one in five general practices in England and Wales found that practices provided most of the routine care for 75% of their diabetic patients. In total, 96% had diabetic registers identifying 1.9% of their patient populations as having diabetes, and 71% held diabetic clinics, of which two-thirds were run by a general practitioner and a nurse, and one-third by a nurse alone. Just over half (54%) shared patient management protocols with the local secondary care team.

Protocol for a diabetic clinic in general practice

Annual assessment[56,80]

One practice that has a well-organised review system[80] arranges a preliminary appointment a week before the annual check at the diabetic review clinic for blood tests. At this time they issue a urine bottle for an early-morning sample of urine and remind patients to bring the sample and records of blood or urine monitoring to the clinic.

The practice shares the care of most patients with type 1 diabetes, alternating with the hospital clinic. Type 2 diabetic patients are usually cared for in the practice unless there are specific problems. The hospital looks after children under 16 years of age and pregnant women.

The protocol for the annual check involves 20 minutes with the practice nurse, who takes the history, performs the examination and gives advice. The nurse instils 0.5% tropicamide eyedrops and measures visual acuity unless the patient is under the care of the hospital eye department. The GP then reviews the history and findings with the nurse and patient, and examines the patient's fundi as appropriate. The computerised data make regular audit very straightforward.

Physical examination at the annual diabetic review

This includes the following:

- body mass index calculation (i.e. weight in kilograms/(height in metres))^2
- blood pressure measurement with the patient sitting and wearing an appropriate-sized cuff
- palpation of pedal and posterior tibial pulses
- measurement of foot sensation by one or more of the following:
    (i) 10-gm monofilament weight (if not detected, sensation is impaired)
    (ii) vibration of 128-Hz tuning fork over the medial malleolus (perception for <5 seconds denotes impaired sensation)
    (iii) assessment of ankle jerk with tendon hammer (this is less reliable in elderly people)
- inspection of feet for colour and temperature, footwear, nail care, callosities, fissures, fungal infection, blisters, ulcers, claw toes, prominent metatarsal heads and Charcot arthropathy
- inspection of injection sites
- visual acuity in corrected state, using standard 6-m (or 3-m) Snellen chart. Use a pin hole if the corrected acuity is <6/9.
- retinal examination by one of the following:
    (i) direct ophthalmology through pupils dilated with 1% tropicamide
    (ii) a combination of direct ophthalmoscopy and slit-lamp biomicroscopy
    (iii) retinal photography through a fixed site or mobile non-mydriatic fundus camera.

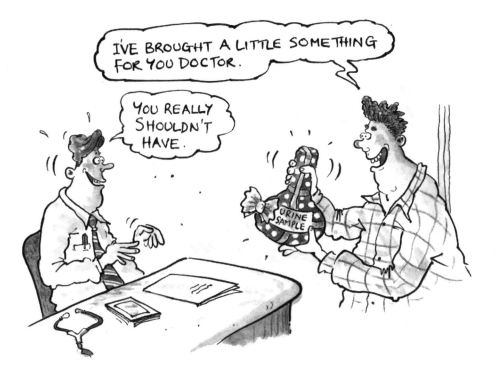

Biochemical analysis at the annual diabetic review

This includes the following:

- dipstick urine analysis for proteinuria (*see* page 85)
- urine testing for microalbuminuria in type 1 diabetes
- blood testing of:
    (i) glycosylated haemoglobin
    (ii) serum creatinine
    (iii) serum total cholesterol and high density lipoprotein cholesterol.

History, advice and education at the annual review

This should include the following:

- smoking history
- effects of diabetes on lifestyle (e.g. the importance of not smoking, dietary limitations)
- review glycaemic control from self-monitoring records and enquire about the frequency of hypo- and hyperglycaemic symptoms
- review the patient's knowledge of 'hypo' management
- education and reinforcement of advice on diet, alcohol consumption, aerobic exercise and lifestyle
- for patients with type 1 diabetes, check the injection technique and rotation of injection sites
- discuss driving, and check that the Driver and Vehicle Licensing Agency (DVLA) has been informed. Reinforce the issue of hypoglycaemia and precautions such as having easily available sugar
- review the patient's treatment, including side-effects and compliance, and check that the patient understands how to take their medication as well as injection site rotation
- assess the patient's knowledge of diabetes and self-management skills, including warning signs for complications (e.g. intermittent claudication, angina pectoris, foot problems). Enquire about any history of chest pains and shortness of breath
- review footwear provision. Enquire about cramps, pins-and-needles sensation, numbness and burning pains. The best care will be provided by primary healthcare teams with a well co-ordinated approach where each member's roles and responsibilities are clear, as described in the example in Box 7.3
- review the need for contact with dietetics, chiropody, orthotics and diabetes specialist nurse support
- enquire about symptoms of neuropathy, and advise on problems of erectile dysfunction in men

- provide pre-pregnancy counselling or contraception advice where appropriate
- check on dental care, free prescriptions and identification cards such as MedicAlert
- calculate and discuss the risk of coronary heart disease and modification of risk factors
- check the patient's knowledge of self-help groups (e.g. Diabetes UK).

Box 7.3 Implementation of guidelines for the assessment of the diabetic foot in the primary care setting[81]

The hospital podiatrist and the diabetes nurse facilitator have ensured the distribution of the guidelines to all practices, as well as presenting them at local conference and study days. Every practice has been offered the opportunity for a teaching and discussion session with the hospital podiatrist. The effectiveness of the guidelines has been evaluated. Benefits identified include increased confidence among nurses in diabetic foot assessment, improved referral quality and improved cross-professional communication.

Treatment targets

These are as follows:

- to maintain blood glucose levels between 4 and 8 mmol/L
- to achieve HbA_{1c} of 7.0 mmol/L or below
- to maintain body mass index at between 20 and 25
- to achieve a blood pressure level of $\leq 140/80$ mmHg.[54,57]

Good practice when looking after teenagers

The SIGN guidelines recommend even closer surveillance of the diabetic state of teenagers than that which is provided for adults with diabetes.[74]

1 Conduct regular screening for risk factors and complications:
   - urinary microalbuminuria excretion twice per year
   - blood pressure and retinal screening annually
   - check smoking status
   - lipids and body mass index.
2 Provide advice on smoking, alcohol and drugs

3 Give information about diabetes in pregnancy and contraceptive advice for all adolescent women
4 Devise a system for contacting defaulters.

Microalbuminuria screening[82]

Patients should provide a mid-stream specimen of the first voided urine in the morning. See the flowchart in Figure 7.1.

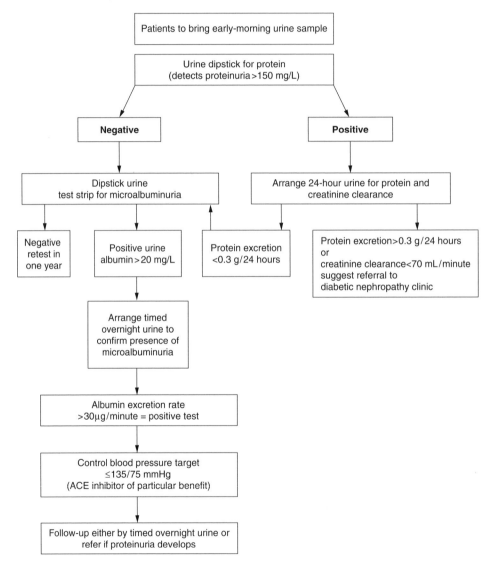

Figure 7.1: Measurement of microalbumin concentration in urine at diabetic annual review (reproduced with permission from Davies S[82]).

Watch out for vulnerable patient groups

People with diabetes who are living in continuing-care homes may not be covered by the practice protocol to the same extent as an able patient who attends the practice's in-house diabetic clinic. Staff turnover and agency staff may disrupt continuity of care and lead to inconsistent practice, as demonstrated in Box 7.4. In nursing homes, residents are becoming increasingly frail and dependent, so realistic targets should be set in partnership with the patient's family and the nursing-home staff.

Box 7.4 Diabetes care in nursing and residential homes[83]

When 75 continuing-care homes were surveyed, researchers found that many residents had diabetes, and that there was a lack of structured care such as monitoring and annual medical reviews within the homes. There was an overwhelming need for staff training and information. Blood glucose monitoring was performed in 81% of nursing homes and only 11% of residential homes. Half of the insulin-treated residents were not monitored. One-third of carers considered that they had access to dietetic advice, 86% to a chiropody service and 73% to ophthalmology. Many staff requested more up-to-date information and education.

Setting outcomes measures for diabetic care

It is really important to agree specific outcome measures when you are setting up your protocol or updating it, so that you can assess how well you are performing and take remedial action as necessary. Box 7.5 gives an outline of the types of outcome measures within which you should fix specific targets or indicators.

Box 7.5 Different perspectives on outcomes of diabetes care[5]

Practice GPs and practice nurses

- Achievement of optimal glucose levels
- Prevention of long-term complications
- Tailoring of regimen to meet the need of the individual

Patients
- Avoidance of short-term complications (e.g. hypoglycaemia)
- Psychosocial needs (e.g. to achieve a balance between health and well-being)
- To be involved in treatment decisions

Reflection exercises

Exercise 13

Undertake an analysis of the strengths, weaknesses, opportunities and threats (SWOT) of the way in which your practice operates its systems and procedures for managing people with diabetes. This will involve convening a group to represent all elements of your practice team (e.g. GP, nurse, manager/support staff, dietitian, podiatrist). You will be considering:

(i) your infrastructure – capacity for computerised recall, the practice protocol, access and availability of diabetes clinics, hardware and software, information resources
(ii) your capability – staff numbers and posts, skills (clinical skills such as more advanced levels of diabetes care, as well as personal and communication skills and information technology)
(iii) your capacity – how you cope with demand
(iv) the extent to which you work as a team across the practice, with others from secondary care or the independent sector, and most of all with patients, including responding to feedback to achieve patient-centred care.

Use the 14 components of clinical governance described in Chapter 1 as a check-list for the SWOT analysis.

Then make a plan for improvement – what you need to learn (and transfer your needs and action plan to your personal and practice development plans), what you need to buy, who you need to appoint or involve and what you need to reorganise.

Exercise 14

Invite the local consultant specialising in diabetes to visit the practice for an in-house educational session. Discuss the last 10 referral letters written to the hospital and the 10 most recent letters from the consultant to the practice. Could you have done more in the practice? Were the responding letters from the hospital staff appropriate? Do they need to learn more about the problems of general practice? Ask the consultant to review your practice protocol and discuss how to provide more seamless care for patients, shifting work and resources to primary care as far as possible.

Invite the local community pharmacists, the dietitian, local optometrists and podiatrist to join you for this educational session, and positively encourage them to contribute to the discussions.

Exercise 15

Conduct an audit of the process of diabetic disease management in your practice, in order to determine the proportion of patients in your practice who are known to have diabetes, who have had an annual review, including BMI, diet review, update on smoking status (and advice given if appropriate), urinanalysis, blood pressure taken and treatment changed accordingly, HbA_{1c}, lipids, creatinine, visual acuity, fundoscopy through dilated pupils, and foot health check.

Exercise 16

Conduct an audit of the outcome of diabetic disease management in your practice, in order to determine the proportion of people with diabetes who have achieved the targets set out in your practice protocol for glycaemic and blood pressure control and other outcome measures, such as the number of hospital admissions for people with diabetes, BMI, smoking status, etc. (*see* Box 5.8).

Now that you have completed these interactive reflection exercises, transfer the information to the relevant section about your learning needs in the empty template on pages 101–10 if you are working on your own personal development plan, or to the practice personal and professional development plan on pages 127–33 if you are working on a practice team learning plan. Don't forget to keep the evidence of your learning in your personal portfolio.

CHAPTER 8

Organising diabetic services in the district

There are wide variations in standards of care for people with diabetes, so that some people with diabetes are more at risk of long-term complications such as blindness, heart disease and kidney disease than others, depending on where they live.[84] For example, half of the health authorities in England do not have district-wide eye screening programmes, two-thirds of hospitals do not know how many of their diabetes patients have received full health checks, and four in ten GP practices do not have guidelines for referring patients with diabetes to secondary care.[34,84]

The general public are unaware of how common diabetes is, or of how serious a disease it is. Therefore one of the tasks for a district or the government is to raise awareness of diabetes among the public, especially for those in high-risk groups.

A recent review of diabetes services urges primary care groups and trusts to review the quality of diabetes care in their constituent general practices. The report recommends commissioning diabetes services from hospitals, employing specialist diabetes nurses, podiatrists, dietitians and other community nursing staff, and working with hospitals to improve services as necessary (e.g. retinal screening if it is not well established).[84] Box 8.1 gives more details.

Box 8.1 The recommendations of the Audit Commission for health authorities, primary care groups/primary care trusts or local health groups (LHGs) in planning services[84]

- Include diabetes as one of the priorities in the health improvement programme to educate the population about risk factors and raise awareness of diabetes, particularly in high-risk groups.
- Establish and maintain population-based information systems, such as registers, to monitor the health of people with diabetes,

including information about health outcomes and investigations, linked to call–recall systems for structured reviews.

- Work with clinical audit colleagues to feed back results to local practices, and encourage joint monitoring across primary and secondary care.
- Monitor processes and outcomes, support necessary change, and consider clinical governance arrangements for diabetes.
- Estimate future demands on services and work using information from the register and other demographic data.
- Identify staffing and monies dedicated to diabetes care, ensuring that there are proper systems in place for managing resources.
- Review patient satisfaction with current services, identify population's needs and review current use of services.
- Review arrangements for out-of-hours support and advice.
- Identify areas where physical access is poor, and develop outreach services and other solutions.
- Ensure the provision of comprehensive district-wide retinal screening.
- Establish and support a Local Diabetes Services Advisory group with multidisciplinary clinical and lay input to identify areas for improvement and promote integrated services from a patient perspective.
- Facilitate ongoing training for GPs, practice nurses and community staff.
- Facilitate the development of clinical guidelines, including guidance about appropriate management by specialist teams and primary care.
- Improve the prevention and early detection of diabetes.
- Improve information for planning and quality control.
- Review resource allocation for diabetes across sectors, and for delivering the National Service Framework.
- Develop, implement and evaluate evidence-based multiprofessional guidelines on the management of people with diabetes.

Services need to be designed from the viewpoint of the user, and tailored to the individual patient. The provision of care for people with chronic diseases, including diabetes, is shifting from secondary to primary care, with the benefits of increased access to care and increased patient satisfaction. Primary care trusts provide an opportunity to reconfigure services around patient needs. More community-based diabetes specialist nurse support is required, as well as community-focused education and support, particularly for practice nurses. The National Service Framework (NSF) and Long-Term Service Agreements (LTSA) will provide the vehicle for a whole-district approach based on the patients' needs if those in the district are committed to this vision.

Box 8.2

One example of good practice cited in the Audit Commission's recent report[84] is a district-wide project organised by Bradford Health Authority. A total of 19 GPs with a specialist interest in diabetes run satellite clinics that are supported by specialist nurses, dietitians and chiropodists. A total of 65 local optometrists are available to undertake annual screening for people with diabetes. Locally agreed guidelines, protocols for treatment and referral work well. The district diabetes register is thought to cover at least 85% of people with diabetes. The achievements in Bradford are all the more impressive as the population of 350 000 is subject to much poverty, deprivation, unemployment and poor housing, with a substantial ethnic minority population from South-East Asia with high rates of diabetes.

District planning groups should consult with one or more relevant consumer groups so that people with diabetes can have greater involvement in the development of their diabetic services.[11]

The key elements to be followed when planning service or health improvements for district residents with diabetes mellitus are shown in Box 8.3.

Box 8.3 Key elements for planning diabetes services or health improvements[5]

- Setting up a multidisciplinary group to exchange ideas, develop partnerships and plan and implement change. At least 60% of health authorities have already set up a Local Diabetes Service Advisory Group (LDSAG) or its equivalent.
- Assessing the healthcare needs of the local population. This would identify problems specific to individual districts, such as a large ethnic minority population, or specific local service issues such as problems with recruiting medical staff.

- Using nationally and internationally available standards to develop and agree the aims and objectives of the local diabetes service and local standards in terms of structure, process and outcome of care.
- Developing local protocols of care, including screening for diabetes, the use of population databases, health promotion, foot care and retinal screening.
- Developing protocols on the management of patients at the primary/secondary care interface.
- Ensuring the training and professional development of those caring for people with diabetes.
- Planning service reconfiguration where appropriate (e.g. the development of outreach clinics).
- Planning evaluation and clinical audit, including economic evaluation.

Population databases

Developments in information technology have enabled more comprehensive databases of diabetes care to be established and used. These have progressed from simple card indices of individuals known to have the disorder to sophisticated electronic databases.

To ensure accuracy when compiling and updating population databases on diabetes, multiple, frequently overlapping sources must be used, including general practices, hospital systems (including the pathology laboratory), health authority data and retinal screening programmes. Guard against duplicate entry if the demographic data are slightly different.

Box 8.4

A report from Sheffield of their experience of compiling a district diabetes register for a population of 307 000 found that input from primary and secondary care was vital for the register to succeed. In total, 64 of 65 practices and all of the hospital diabetes clinics participated. General practices checked lists of people with diabetes known to the hospitals from their clinic and laboratory records. The resulting register identified 5185 individuals as having diabetes. Data from hospital and laboratory sources missed 635 people with diabetes who were known only to general practices, and 425 people with diabetes who were known to hospital and laboratory sources but not included on the practice's own diabetes registers. The prevalence of diabetes that was recorded was 1.84%.[85]

There is likely to be an underestimate of the number of people with diabetes, especially those treated with dietary therapy alone.

In most places where such databases exist, individuals with diabetes are largely ignorant of the fact that their demographic and clinical details are held in this form, in addition to the clinical record. Permission should be sought from the patient in line with the Data Protection Act. It is important to seek advice from your local Caldicott guardian.

Box 8.5 Epidemiological information that is needed for healthcare needs assessments of individuals with diabetes in a local area

- The number of individuals with clinically diagnosed diabetes in a given population (the *prevalence*)
- The number of new patients who require diagnosis, stabilisation and programmes of education and long-term care (the *incidence*)
- The number of individuals who have, or are likely to develop, specific complications

---

Integrated care pathways (ICP)

The numbers of guidelines being published by national bodies such as NICE, the special interest organisations, and the continuing work of SIGN in Scotland mean that there is sometimes a lack of consensus between the guidelines, with resulting confusion for practitioners.

Integrated care pathways may not only achieve more uniform clinical care, but also help with more efficient use of resources, as in the example given in Box 8.6. The local working group that is producing the draft integrated care pathway (ICP) should reflect all those with an interest, including patients' representatives. There should be a great deal of consultation in order to achieve maximum local ownership of the pathway and associated guidelines.

Box 8.6 Integrated care pathway associated with a reduction in diabetes non-attenders from 19% to 1%[86]

The 'did not attend' (DNA) rate for new patient diabetes appointments in St Helens & Knowsley was high (15%, or 201 of 1336 patients for 1996–98). This study examined the impact of an integrated care pathway on DNA rates. The two elements of the ICP that were designed to impact upon DNAs were very successful: (1) a detailed information pack sent to patients with their appointment and (2) a telephone call one week before their appointment. Sending patients an information pack and telephoning them a week before their appointment reduced DNAs to almost zero.

The NSF for diabetes will guide the development of local services.

Box 8.7 An online Web-based educational and clinical resource for the management of patients with diabetes[87]

The Tayside Regional Diabetes Network has developed a web-based resource to support regional diabetes care in Tayside, Scotland. The process involved:

- developing locally agreed, region-wide protocols derived from national evidence-based guidelines
- defining management plans for the care of patients with diabetes and its complications
- providing comprehensive details of local staff, diabetes services and clinics
- incorporating a patient resource, including information leaflets.

A multidisciplinary team produced the material, integrating regionally agreed protocols, educational materials, automated audit and decision support text, to provide online NHSnet access for the regional care of people with diabetes.
See www.diabetes-healthnet.ac.uk

Measures of process

Recommendations for the audit of diabetes services include the following:[5]

1 average waiting times in diabetic clinics
2 average time spent with the doctor, nurse or other health worker
3 quality of communication with the primary care team
4 the frequency with which the following are recorded in the clinical notes:
   • body weight
   • state of optic fundi (observed through dilated pupils) and visual acuity
   • blood pressure
   • urinary albumin concentration
   • percentage of glycosylated haemoglobin
   • serum cholesterol (total and high-density-lipoprotein (HDL) cholesterol)
   • state of injection sites (in insulin-treated patients)
   • state of the feet
   • presence of peripheral pulses.

Measures of outcome

The outcomes of diabetes care to be measured at primary care organisation (PCO) or district level can be formulated from the aims and objectives that are agreed as part of the local health improvement programme.

The following six indicators might be used by a district on a routine basis:[5]

• the prevalence of clinically diagnosed diabetes
• the number of patients who have had at least one hypoglycaemic emergency within the last year that required therapeutic intervention by a health professional, expressed as a proportion of the population known to have diabetes
• the number of patients who have had at least one hyperglycaemic emergency within the last year that required hospital admission, expressed as a proportion of the population of patients known to have diabetes

- the standard mortality rate (SMR) for death due to diabetes mellitus
- the number of years of life lost per 10 000 resident population by death due to diabetes mellitus
- the number of years of life lost by death due to diabetes mellitus.

Knowing the population denominator of people with diabetes is crucial for the calculation of these indicators. A few districts have comprehensive diabetes population databases, but most will have to extrapolate from published estimates of prevalence.

Diabetes centres

The main components of diabetes services are the hospital-based diabetes team or teams (usually one or more consultant diabetologists (or a paediatrician), other consultant staff, a specialist nurse, dietitian and podiatrist, with suitable junior medical, laboratory and administrative support), the primary care team (general practitioner, practice nurse and administrative support) and other community support (podiatrist, dietitian and community nurse). About 75% of districts or their equivalent have a 'diabetes centre'.[5,88,89]

Ideally, diabetes centres should (and some do) provide the hub of the local diabetes services, and a place where patients and their carers, as well as staff from the hospital and community, can meet. They offer clinical advice and education on diabetes to all on a single site where most of the professional and social services required are accessible. In many cases their operational philosophy and organisation take into account the special bridging role between specialist and primary care diabetes services.

Diabetes centres should offer some or all of the following facilities:[89]

- education services for patients and their carers, staff working in the centre and professionals from primary and secondary care
- an agreed educational curriculum for each group
- facilities for clinical advice and regular review, including the annual review
- drop-in access for people with diabetic problems
- referrals for further diagnosis and treatment of diabetes
- joint clinics with ophthalmologists, nephrologists and other specialists
- dietary advice, including information, teaching and review by specialist dietitians

- chiropody advice, education and treatment
- psychological and social advice and treatment
- a flexible outreach service
- a 24-hour telephone helpline
- a secure and effective computerised information system
- a venue for the audit of local diabetes services
- a place to house and update the diabetes register
- a meeting place for primary and secondary care staff to hold joint clinical meetings
- a focus for integrated care, providing the opportunity to create individualised programmes of care for people, which are sufficiently flexible to meet their changing needs through a lifetime with diabetes
- the opportunity for people with diabetes to obtain all or a large part of the services that are relevant to diabetes care in one place
- a children's play area
- a place where people with diabetes and their families can meet and share their problems, experiences and solutions (e.g. local Diabetes UK branch meetings)
- a place where other meetings relevant to diabetes can be held (e.g. Local Diabetes Services Advisory Group (LDSAG) meetings
- a place where advice can be given to groups of people with special needs related to diabetes (e.g. children, young adults, pre-pregnancy counselling).

Referral criteria

Referral criteria should be clear, as discussed by the LDSAG, and disseminated through educational events and guidelines within districts. Some of the key criteria relate to the following:

- diabetes in childhood, which is urgent if newly diagnosed
- type 1 diabetes
- consider referral of newly diagnosed type 2 diabetes for initial assessment, target agreement and exclusion of secondary causes
- pregnancy
- problems relating to therapeutic targets and complications
- significant vomiting or ketonuria that requires urgent advice, as do cases of 'hot foot' and sudden visual loss.

Remember that it is important to agree discharge criteria too, for those patients who no longer need to be seen by the hospital team.

Reflection exercise

Exercise 17

Find out if there are any district-wide guidelines for diabetes in your area if you don't know already. Ask the local consultants specialising in diabetes or renal medicine, the public health department or the medical audit advisory group (if it still exists or has evolved into another quality body). Compare your practice protocol, including referral criteria and any audit of your practice performance, with the district guidelines or outcome data. How do you match up? Do you, your practice team or those leading on diabetes in the district have any learning needs?

Now that you have completed this interactive reflection exercise, transfer the information to the relevant section about your learning needs in the empty template on pages 101–10 if you are working on your own personal development plan, or to the practice personal and professional development plan on pages 127–33 if you are working on a practice team learning plan. Don't forget to keep the evidence of your learning in your personal portfolio.

CHAPTER 9

Draw up and apply your personal development plan

Although you will probably want to focus on the clinical management of diabetes, you may be interested in making improving your IT skills a focus of your personal development plan (PDP). A PDP on information technology could supplement a practice professional development plan (PPDP) on diabetes (*see* Chapter 10). Therefore we have included a worked example of a personal development plan focused around information technology on pages 111–23.

As we explained in the introduction, you may decide to allocate 50% of the time you intend to spend drawing up and applying a personal development plan in any one year on learning more about diabetes. That would leave space in your learning plan for other important topics such as mental health, coronary heart disease or cancer – whatever is a priority for you, your practice team and your patient population. There will be some overlap between topics. For example, you cannot consider a person with diabetes in isolation from their cardiovascular risk factors, and that means understanding and knowing how to prevent and manage cardiovascular problems, too.

The example given is very comprehensive, and you may not want to include so much detail in your own personal development plan. You might include different topics and educational activities because your needs and circumstances are different to those of the example practitioner here. Alternatively, you might move on to Chapter 10 and modify the example of a practice professional development plan shown there to your personal development plan.

Transfer the information about your learning needs from any of the reflection exercises at the end of the chapters that are relevant to you and that you have completed to the empty template of the personal development plan that follows on pages 101–10. The reflection exercises you decide to select will depend on the focus of your personal development plan – diabetes, or IT (as in the worked example here).

The conclusions you have drawn at the end of each exercise will feature in the action plan of your personal development plan. Some more ideas about the preliminary information you should be gathering for your personal development plan are given in the boxes of the template.

Template for your personal development plan

What topic have you chosen?

Who chose it?

Justify why this topic is a priority:
a personal or professional priority?

a practice priority?

a district priority?

a national priority?

Who will be included in your personal development plan?
(Anyone other than you? Other GPs, employed staff, attached staff, others from outside the practice, patients?)

What baseline information will you collect and how?

How will you identify your learning needs?
(How will you obtain this and who will do it? Self-completion check-lists, discussion, appraisal, audit, patient feedback?)

What are the learning needs of the practice and how do they match your needs?

Is there any patient or public input to your personal development plan?

Aims of your personal development plan arising from the preliminary data-gathering exercise:

How might you integrate the 14 components of clinical governance into your personal development plan, focusing on the topic of . . . . ?

Establishing a learning culture:

Managing resources and services:

Establishing a research and development culture:

Reliable and accurate data:

Evidence-based practice and policy:

Confidentiality:

Health gain:

Coherent team:

Audit and evaluation:

Meaningful involvement of patients and the public:

Health promotion:

Risk management:

Accountability and performance:

Core requirements:

Action plan (include objectives, timetabled action and expected outcomes)

How does your personal development plan tie in with your other strategic plans? (For example, the practice's business or development plan, the Primary Care Investment Plan or health improvement programme)

What additional resources will you require to execute your plan and from where do you hope to obtain them?
(Will you have to pay any course fees? Will you be able to organise any protected time for learning in working hours?)

How will you evaluate your personal development plan?

How will you know when you have achieved your objectives?
(How will you measure success?)

How will you disseminate the learning from your plan to the rest of the practice team and patients? How will you sustain your new-found knowledge or skills?

How will you handle new learning requirements as they crop up?

Check out whether the topic you choose to learn is a priority and the way in which you plan to learn about it is appropriate. Photocopy this pro forma for future use.

Your topic:

How have you identified your learning need(s)?

(a) PCO requirement ☐   (e) Appraisal need ☐

(b) Practice business ☐   (f) New to post ☐
plan

(c) Legal mandatory ☐   (g) Individual decision ☐
requirement

(d) Job requirement ☐   (h) Patient feedback ☐

(i) Other ☐

. . . .

Have you discussed or planned your learning needs with anyone else?

Yes ☐   No ☐   If yes, who?

. . . .

What are the learning need(s) and/or objective(s) in terms of the following?

Knowledge. What new information do you hope to gain to help you to do this?

. . . .

Skills. What should you be able to do differently as a result of undertaking this learning in your development plan?

. . . .

Behaviour/professional practice. How will this impact on the way in which you subsequently do things?

. . . .

Details and date of desired development activity:

. . . .

Details of any previous training and/or experience you have in this area/dates:

. . . .

What is your current performance in this area compared to the requirements of your job?

Need significant development in this area ☐	Need some development in this area ☐
Satisfactory in this area ☐	Do well in this area ☐

What is the level of job relevance that this area has to your role and responsibilities?

Has no relevance to job ☐	Has some relevance ☐
Relevant to job ☐	Very relevant ☐
Essential to job ☐	

Describe what aspect of your job it is relevant to, and how the proposed education/training is relevant:

. . . .

Do you need additional support in identifying a suitable development activity?

Yes ☐   No ☐

What do you need?

. . . .

Describe the differences or improvements for you, your practice, PCO and/or employing NHS trust as a result of undertaking this activity:

. . . .

Assess the priority of your proposed educational/training activity:

Urgent ☐   High ☐   Medium ☐   Low ☐

Describe how the proposed activity will meet your learning needs rather than any other type of course or training on the topic:

. . . .

If you had a free choice would you want to learn this?

Yes/No

If **No**, why not? (please circle all that apply):

Waste of time
I have already done it
It is not relevant to my work or career goals
Other

If **Yes**, what reasons are most important to you? (put them in rank order):

To improve my performance
To increase my knowledge
To get promotion
I am just interested in it
To be better than my colleagues
To do a more interesting job
To enable me to be more confident
Because it will help me

Record of your learning

Write in the topic, date, time spent and type of learning

	Activity 1	Activity 2	Activity 3	Activity 4
In-house formal learning				
External courses				
Informal and personal				
Qualifications and/or experience gained				

Worked example of a personal development plan: information technology (IT)

Who chose it? It might be your own choice or that of someone in the practice team or PCO who thinks that you should have additional skills in IT.

Justify why the topic is a priority:

(i) *a personal or professional priority?* You may have chosen IT because you see a need for it yourself or as an inevitable development in your work. You may have agreed as part of your work development, or as a requirement of a change in work duties or responsibilities. You may have volunteered after development in IT was identified as a practice or PCG/PCT need.

(ii) *a practice priority?* Perhaps the practice has identified that you have not been entering data about people with diabetes, or that the practice annual report would be easier to prepare if everyone entered data in a consistent way. You may want to introduce a computerised patient-call system for people with diabetes. The practice may want to use IT for another project or for audit, but has insufficient IT skills available, or the practice may be preparing to become 'paperless'. Patient need may have increased the number of computerised protocols in use. The practice may have a need for an in-house expert in hardware or software to reduce support bills.

(iii) *a district priority?* The PCO may need more data than can be supplied by paper records, or they may need additional expertise. Electronic links with health authorities and hospital trusts are becoming increasingly important (e.g. in the maintenance of a district diabetic register). The health authority may have a commitment to have all practices connected to NHSnet within a certain time framework, and a Local Implementation Strategy that includes other IT projects.

(iv) *a national priority?* The government wants to see all practices connected to the NHSnet. It wants you to be able to communicate with secondary care for quicker transmission of patient information and for making appointments at the time when the patient is referred. It expects health professionals to be able to take advantage of the Internet opportunities for retrieval of up-to-date information. The National Service Framework for diabetes will be easier to implement if the NHS has a good IT infrastructure.

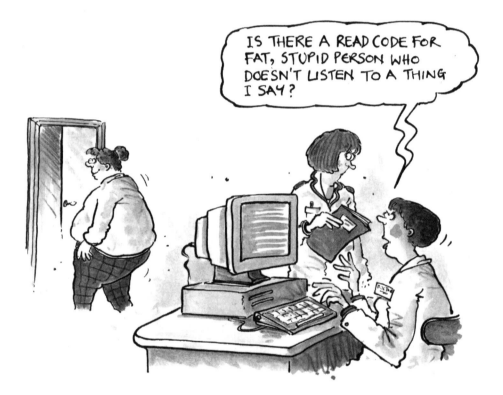

Who will be included in your personal development plan?

You might like to find others who want to increase their skills. Working together or as a cascade of learning from each other makes learning more cost-effective and standardisation of data entry is improved (provided that you do not pass on faulty habits!). Learning skills and then passing them on makes for more effective learning for you, too.

Everyone needs to have the opportunity – reception staff, practice manager, secretaries, *all* of the health professionals, and anyone who is going to enter anything on your computer system. You might want to offer computer-based health information to patients as well, or use patients as a resource. Remember confidentiality and security issues.

You may want to consider IT training as a PCO activity to ensure consistency, exchange skills and reduce costs. Bringing in outside experts in IT training then becomes more cost-effective and can be tailored to the particular needs of the learning group.

Who will collect the baseline information and how?

You could ask the practice manager or secretary, or the IT lead at the PCO, or the health authority IT adviser to find out details of the IT training available. If you are already Internet connected, you can search for other more distant information yourself. You may have a useful health informatics department at a local university or based at a hospital trust. Your computer supplier may provide training (your data-entry clerk may know about this).

You need to know what computer systems are being used in the workplace. The PCO or health authority may already have collected this information.

Find out from the IT adviser what is in the pipeline for the immediate and long-term future development of IT in your area.

How will you identify your learning needs?

Use the check-lists in the earlier sections of this book. Among other methods, you might want to do a SWOT analysis:

Strengths: Enthusiasm. A logical mind. Willingness to go on learning (IT changes rapidly). Communication skills and inter-professional relationships to enable inter-disciplinary working. Organisational and teaching skills. Research skills to provide a resource for IT once learned. User-friendly and well-designed software and hardware in the practice, with sufficient spare capacity for quality improvements.

Opportunities: A relative or friend with IT skills, an in-practice expert, a recent IT learner who is keen to pass on his or her newly acquired knowledge. Expertise at home computing on which you can build for professional proficiency. A decision to gain a qualification in IT, finding a local course of interest, or discovering that NVQ or Microsoft Certification courses are available.

Weaknesses and threats: Deficiencies in equipment, software or availability of training. Other commitments, antagonism or lack of support from others.

You might include a survey of the equipment and software available in your PCO and elsewhere, and list the present competencies of other staff. What levels of expertise are accessible inside and outside your own workplace?

What are the learning needs for the practice and how do they match your needs?

A prioritising exercise as part of drawing up the PDP should have already given you some information. Consider inviting people to express their concerns and opinions at a practice team meeting, or ask another member of staff to organise it. Various members of the practice team might have prioritised IT as a learning need for themselves. The practice manager could ask people to complete a check-list of their own needs and wishes for IT, and what they would like from others.

You might wish to specialise and become an accredited software or hardware expert. Does this fit with the requirements of the practice (or PCO)? Would it be more cost-effective to buy in such expertise?

A GP might wish to become the IT adviser for the health authority or the lead for IT in the PCO. What implications does this have for the practice in terms of cover for clinical sessions?

A secretary may wish to have paid time to go on a computer skills course in order to learn spreadsheet and database skills. Do you already have someone at a lower grade who can do this, or would it free up practice nurse or GP time if she took over some of the data management for audits, etc.?

Providing e-mail or Internet access in the common-room could encourage people to use the computers more. The practice professional development plan might prioritise your extra IT capability as a particular benefit to the practice, depending on what expertise is already there and the extent of your learning needs.

Is there any patient or public input to your plan?

If you are intending to become 'paperless', what do your patients think about it? Do you know what they think about where the screen is in the consulting-room? Do they want to see what you are entering? Do they have concerns about who will access the information and the level of confidentiality, especially if you are taking part in a PCO-wide information-gathering exercise with externally employed audit assistants? How will they be reassured about the collection of data for the PCO's management functions?

Do your patients want to be involved in designing information on health matters? Do they want you to have a website? How do you manage general public enquiries to a practice website? Do they want the development of electronic transmission of prescriptions to the pharmacist of their choice? Do they want to email their prescription requests to you? Would patient-held electronic medical records be acceptable?

Discuss the use of computers at the reception desk. Are there confidentiality issues that concern patients?

Do patients want to use computer programs for health advice or for treatment of, for example, psychological problems? (Cognitive therapy is available as a computer program.)

What mechanism(s) will you use to find out the answers in a meaningful way (not just from the most opinionated or compliant patients)? You may need to think deeply about the reliability of any method, and how representative individual patients are of your whole practice population.[10]

Aims of personal development arising from the preliminary data-gathering exercise

To develop sufficient IT skills to achieve the standards and milestones in the National Service Framework for diabetes as relevant to primary care. To learn, for example, how to:

- use the computer for consulting and prescribing
- set up an appointment and call system and use the system for health promotion messages
- enter Read codes consistently for diabetes mellitus and other diseases
- do a search and audit and use a spreadsheet
- use e-mail and the Internet
- sort out bugs in the software
- use linking with the health authority and hospital trust for

registration, claims and clinical information downloads, and updating of the district's diabetic register
- set up forms for automating referrals, management and activity reports, annual report information, etc.
- set up protocols and guidelines for delegation and consistent recording
- use financial management
- produce patient leaflets and a newsletter
- become 'paperless'.

How might you integrate the 14 components of clinical governance into your personal development plan focusing on the topic of information technology?

Establishing a learning culture: hold regular meetings on different aspects of IT, including 'hands-on' practice for team members to learn new skills and information.

Managing resources and services: identify whether the computer system is being used to its best capacity, ensuring that service contracts are maintained and are cost-effective.

Establishing a research and development culture: a 'Web night', perhaps, to wet people's appetites for searching for health information, using searches to find information, and finding out what is being done elsewhere.

Reliable and accurate data: enter data once, consistently and correctly, be able to retrieve it for a variety of uses and be able to compare the data with others.

Evidence-based practice and policy: find out which systems are accredited for use in general practice. Discover the best methods of sending information between computers.

Confidentiality: ensure that passwords are used correctly and securely and that the data is protected against unauthorised access and not passed to others without knowing the degree of confidentiality with which it will be treated. Screens should only be visible to those who need to read them, and information on patients should not be visible to others.

Health gain: more reliable and accessible data means better quality management and more pro-active care, such as call and recall systems.

Coherent team: everyone needs to know how to enter data consistently and to retrieve that part of it which they require for patient management.

Audit and evaluation: check that there is consistent entry of Read codes, follow the management of specific conditions, and search and audit care in a multiplicity of ways.

Meaningful involvement of patients and the public: use the computer to provide health information requested by patients or to provide an interchange of ideas (e.g. in a newsletter written by both patients and staff). Use computer health education or treatment packages, or just use the computer to provide a randomised stratified selection of patients for your patient focus groups to discuss patient care and services for diabetes.

Health promotion: target health promotion with specific reminders on screen, or select specific groups for action (e.g. to offer assistance with smoking cessation to people with diabetes).

Risk management: Ensure that there are up-to-date records on everything, from the patients to staff qualifications (e.g. last cardiopulmonary resuscitation update), to when the steriliser was last serviced. Reminders for action can be set, and interactions of drugs or allergies recorded.

Accountability and performance: your system must have an 'audit trail' to be accredited (i.e. there must be a record of who entered what and when). Ensure that everyone knows that they must only log on as themselves and why!

Core requirements: could you work out a better skill mix in your practice team to provide more cost-effective computer use?

Action plan (include the objectives above, timetabled action and expected outcomes)

Who is involved? All identified staff who need to learn IT skills with you.

Where? Identify the sites at which training and learning will take place.

Timetabled action: Start date:

By 3 months: preliminary data gathered and staff involved identified.
• Skills that are already present (in practice, in the PCO, health authority, etc.).
• Equipment and systems that are available (your own, the practice, the PCO, outside in a training venue).

- Training that can be obtained (to match your needs).
- Training that could take place (in practice, other practice(s), at college or university, at a commercial IT facility, distance learning, other local or distant venue).
- How it could be done (individual or group, tutor-led or cascade learning).

By 4 months: review current performance.
- Are your skills being utilised in the best way?
- Does the equipment meet the specifications for the tasks that you are required to perform now and those that you anticipate performing in the immediate future?

By 6 months: identify solutions and associated learning needs.
- Arrange the necessary training.
- Make a business plan for any associated equipment needs.
- Arrange cover for yourself and any other staff who are involved to provide protected time for learning.
- Clarify who does what and when.
- Negotiate changes necessary at practice meeting(s).

By 12 months: make the changes.
- Implement the new IT systems or procedures.
- Obtain feedback from other staff about its impact.
- Iron out any difficulties.
- Identify any gaps in the provision.

Expected outcomes: reliable accurate data that is easily entered and retrieved, ease of use, quicker access to records, better quality of care for patients, better access to care for patients, relevant inter-disciplinary shared information, increased safety and security (depending on the exact project carried out).

How does your personal development plan tie in with your other strategic plans? (e.g. the practice's business or development plan, the Primary Care Investment Plan or the health improvement programme)

Development of IT will be an integral part of your practice business or practice personal and professional development plans and of your PCO plans. Make sure that your objectives mesh with theirs.

What additional resources will you require to execute your plan and from where do you hope to obtain them?

Your entitlement to reimbursement of course fees, etc., will depend on your contract and on the priority value that the practice or PCO puts on your development plan to meet their own needs.

The need for any additional equipment will have to be decided on the same basis.

How will you evaluate your learning plan?

Look at the methods that you used to identify your learning needs. How does it all fit? Can you repeat a measure that you adopted to establish your learning needs to determine how much you have learned or the extent to which your performance has improved?

How will you know when you have achieved your objectives?

You will be able to carry out the tasks that you have set yourself, or you will have implemented the changes specified in your objectives list.

How will you disseminate the learning from the plan to the rest of the practice team and patients? How will you sustain your new-found knowledge or skills?

You could let everyone know in a practice newsletter, or let the staff know what has been achieved, or what is now available, at team meetings.

Pass on your skills to other people in the team as required, and keep using your skills to provide information or better structure or systems to your computer programs. You could run an in-house training session to teach others in the practice team how to do one of the new procedures you have mastered.

How will you handle new learning requirements as they crop up?

Keep a record as they arise so that you can consider them later, or add them in if it is essential to do so at this stage.

Check out whether the topic you choose to learn is a priority and the way in which you plan to learn about it is appropriate.

Your topic: *Information Technology*

How have you identified your learning need(s)?

(*a*) PCO requirement	☒	(*e*) Appraisal need	☐
(*b*) Practice business plan	☒	(*f*) New to post	☐
(*c*) Legal mandatory requirement	☐	(*g*) Individual decision	☐
(*d*) Job requirement	☒	(*h*) Patient feedback	☐
		(*i*) Other	☐

Have you discussed or planned your learning needs with anyone else?

Yes ☒ No ☐ If yes, who? *Other staff; PCO IT lead.*

What are the learning need(s) and/or objective(s) in terms of the following?

Knowledge: What new information do you hope to gain to help you to do this?

To learn how to enter data consistently and reliably and how to retrieve information in a useful form.

Skills: What should you be able to do differently as a result of undertaking this learning in your development plan?

Produce the annual report quickly; produce information about workload and services provided by the practice; identify problems with targets at an early stage.

Behaviour/professional practice: How will this impact on the way in which you subsequently do things?

I might be able to improve the quality of information, to improve the delivery of services and to ensure that all income due for item-of-service claims is obtained.

Details and date of desired development activity:

Within three months: attend sessions on use of the software available on the computer system and Read coding. Within six months: start to produce rolling reports on the services, workload and targets.

Details of any previous training and/or experience you have in this area/dates:

Piecemeal self-instruction without structure or specific objectives.

What is your current performance in this area compared to the requirements of your job?

Need significant development in this area	☒	Need some development in this area	☐
Satisfactory in this area	☐	Do well in this area	☐

What is the level of job relevance that this area has to your role and responsibilities?

Has no relevance to job	☐	Has some relevance	☐
Relevant to job	☐	Very relevant	☒
Essential to job	☐		

Describe what aspect of your job it is relevant to, and how the proposed education/training is relevant:

Integral part of my work evaluating and monitoring the performance of the practice team.

Do you need additional support in identifying a suitable development activity?

Yes ☒   No ☐

What do you need?

To know when and where relevant sessions of training are being held. Help in preparing reports.

Describe the differences or improvements for you, your practice, PCO and/or employing NHS trust as a result of undertaking this activity:

I will be able to evaluate the standards of care, monitor performance and assess progress towards targets set by the practice team and PCG. It will be easier to produce the annual report and other information required for outside bodies (e.g. when the practice is assessed).

Assess the priority of your proposed educational/training activity:

Urgent ☐   High ☒   Medium ☐   Low ☐

Describe how the proposed activity will meet your learning needs rather than any other type of course or training on the topic:

The mix of learning from sessions with an experienced user of the software and personal learning by observing others' practice in different settings should help me to identify what I don't know and meet my learning needs.

If you had a free choice would you want to learn this?   <u>Yes</u>/No

If **No**, why not? (please circle all that apply):

Waste of time
I have already done it
It is not relevant to my work or career goals
Other

If **Yes**, what reasons are most important to you? (put them in rank order):

To improve my performance	1
To increase my knowledge	2
To get promotion	
I am just interested in it	
To be better than my colleagues	
To do a more interesting job	
To enable me to be more confident	3
Because it will help me	4

Record of your learning about Information Technology

You would add the date, length of time spent, etc., for each learning activity

	Activity 1 – knowledge of best practice in the use of the software	Activity 2 – learning skills in Read code and other consistent data entry techniques	Activity 3 – learning skills in information retrieval and producing reports	Activity 4 – learning how to impart the skills gained to others in the practice
In-house formal learning				Protected time for other practice team members to learn consistent data entry and the reasons for it
External courses	Sessions with experienced users of the computer software	Read coding course; sessions with experienced users in users group	Attendance at local course on use of Excel and producing reports	A distance-learning course on teaching computer skills
Informal and personal	Sit in with audit clerk and practice manager to discover what their information needs are	Discussion and standardisation agreements with others in the computer users group and other practices in the PCO	Practice information retrieval and report production	Informal sessions whenever a problem is presented; help offered to others as required; informal discussions about harmonisation of data entry
Qualifications and/or experience gained	Experiences of others at the sessions; gain experience in use	Experience and practice in techniques	Reports produced and available for the practice team and PCO or for outside bodies such as the health authority	Monitoring of data entered and audit of standards. Certificate of completion of course

CHAPTER 10

Draw up and apply your practice personal and professional development plan

The *practice personal and professional development plan (PPDP)* should cater for everyone who works in a practice. Clinical governance principles will balance the development needs of the population, the practice, the PCO *and* your individual *personal development plan (PDP)*.

You might want to start by identifying your own learning needs, combining them with those of other people and then checking them against the practice business plan. You could start from the other direction – develop a practice-based personal and professional development plan from your business plan and then identify your individual learning needs within that. Whichever direction you start from, you must ensure that you integrate your individual needs with those of your practice and the needs and directives of the NHS.

Your learning plan should complement the professional development of other individuals and of the practice. If you are working on a project that involves change for other people as well as yourself, it is better to work together towards a common goal and co-ordinate multiprofessional learning across traditional boundaries.

If you work in a number of different roles or posts, gaps and duplication of activities should be avoided. After reflection about the boundaries between your roles, you may be able to focus your learning so that meeting your needs in one role benefits another.

Make your learning plan flexible. You may want to add something in later when circumstances suddenly change or an additional need becomes apparent, perhaps as a result of a complaint or hearing something new at a meeting.

Long-term locums (say, longer than six months), assistants, retained doctors and salaried GPs should all be included in the practice plan. Remember to include all of those staff who work for the practice, however few their hours – you cannot manage without them or they would not be there!

Time is one of the resources that must be considered when drawing up your action plan. Adequate resources must be in place for your learning needs, and protected time must be built in.

Template for your practice personal and professional development plan

What topic have you chosen?

Who chose it?

Justify why this topic is a priority:

a personal or professional priority?

a practice priority?

a district priority?

a national priority?

Who will be included in your practice personal and professional development plan?
(Anyone other than you? Other GPs, employed staff, attached staff, others from outside the practice, patients?)

What baseline information will you collect and how?

How will you identify your learning needs?
(How will you obtain this and who will do it? Self-completion check-lists, discussion, appraisal, audit, patient feedback?)

What are the learning needs of the practice and how do they match individuals' needs?

Is there any patient or public input to your practice personal and professional development plan?

Aims of your practice-based plan arising from the preliminary data-gathering exercise:

How might you integrate the 14 components of clinical governance into your practice personal and professional development plan, focusing on the topic of . . . . ?

Establishing a learning culture:

Managing resources and services:

Establishing a research and development culture:

Reliable and accurate data:

Evidence-based practice and policy:

Confidentiality:

Health gain:

Coherent team:

Audit and evaluation:

Meaningful involvement of patients and the public:

Health promotion:

Risk management:

Accountability and performance:

Core requirements:

Action plan (include objectives, timetabled action and expected outcomes)

How does your practice personal and professional development plan tie in with your other strategic plans? (For example, the practice's business or development plan, the Primary Care Investment Plan or the health improvement programme)

What additional resources will you require to execute your plan and from where do you hope to obtain them?
(Will you have to pay any course fees? Will you be able to organise any protected time for learning in working hours?)

How will you evaluate your practice personal and professional development plan?

How will you know when you have achieved your objectives?
(How will you measure success?)

How will you disseminate the learning from your plan to the rest of the practice team and patients? How will you sustain your new-found knowledge or skills?

How will you handle new learning requirements as they crop up?

Record of your learning

Write in the topic, date, time spent and type of learning

	Activity 1	Activity 2	Activity 3	Activity 4
In-house formal learning				
External courses				
Informal and personal				
Qualifications and/or experience gained				

Worked example of a practice personal and professional development plan: diabetes mellitus

Who chose the topic? Many of the practice team may realise that improving the care of people with diabetes is of overriding importance to be able to meet the standards and milestones of the National Service Framework (NSF) for diabetes.

Justify why the topic is a priority:

(i) *a practice and professional priority?* Good risk management is an essential part of diabetic care both at a clinical level for individuals with diabetes, and from an organisational perspective when identifying new cases and monitoring their continuing care. Therefore investing time and effort in improving the care of those with diabetes should produce tangible and significant health gains for individual patients.

(ii) *a district priority?* Districts are working with PCOs to implement the NSFs for diabetes and coronary heart disease and provide more effective primary and secondary prevention for those with diabetes.

(iii) *a national priority?* The cost of medical complications in diabetic patients is high. Effective diabetic management is cost-effective to the NHS, through avoiding complications and keeping those with diabetes at work, as well as maintaining their health and well-being. Diabetes is a national priority, as it is the subject of a National Service Framework.

Who will be included in the practice-based personal and professional development plan?

You might include:

- GPs
- practice nurses
- health visitors
- district nurses
- diabetic liaison nurse from local NHS trust
- optometrist
- community pharmacist
- chiropodist or podiatrist
- practice manager

- reception staff
- Diabetes UK representative
- patients with diabetes, and their families.

Who will collect the baseline information and how?

A receptionist/computer operator could do an electronic search in your practice to identify patients with diabetes if appropriately coded. Otherwise it will be laborious to set up a diabetic disease register from paper records, repeat prescriptions, recall, etc. Once you know who your diabetic patients are, you can audit their care and see what you need to learn.

The local public health department at your health authority should be able to supply data about morbidity and mortality rates in your district. They may also have national data on file about the average numbers per 1000 population who might be expected to have diabetes, categorised according to age, gender, ethnic group, etc., or you can obtain this information from your local medical library.

The local hospital trust could give you routine and acute data about referrals and admissions of patients with diabetes. The hospital audit department may have undertaken work on diabetes and might give you a breakdown of results identifying your patient or PCO populations.

Where are you now?

- Establish how many people with diabetes you have identified in your patient population, and whether they are types 1 or 2.
- Compare your practice protocol for managing diabetes with a protocol cited in the literature as 'best practice' or a recommended district protocol or guideline. If you do not have a practice protocol, write one or adopt someone else's.
- Look at how many individuals attend follow-up appointments in line with your practice protocol – for the various groups with diabetes, different age groups or ethnic groups. Determine whether you may need to make follow-up appointments more available or convenient.
- Determine how good glucose control is in your patients with diabetes. How many have good control with an HbA_{1c} of $<6.5\%$? How many are borderline at HbA_{1c} 6.5–7.5%? How many have poor control $>7.5\%$?
- Focus on prevention of risks, such as looking at the number of individuals who smoke, are overweight, or have a history of coronary heart disease.
- Review the extent of education or training that the clinical staff have received about diabetes.

- Undertake an analysis of the strengths, weaknesses, opportunities and threats (SWOT) in relation to diabetes, with your practice team.

What information will you obtain about individual learning wishes and needs?

You might review the practice protocol and baseline information with as many staff as possible at a discussion group and find out whether they feel competent as individuals to carry out their roles and responsibilities, or whether they want to realign their duties. They might comment on how well others are fulfilling their responsibilities and suggest improvements to the systems or procedures that have educational and resource consequences, such as training sessions, new equipment, or effects on other parts of the practice organisation.

A significant event audit such as whether a person with diabetes becomes blind or has a leg amputated, or someone under 60 years of age with diabetes has a myocardial infarction, might reveal the learning needs of individuals and practice systems.

What are the learning needs of the practice and how do they match the needs of the individual?

Responding to the queries from the district or PCO about the practice's diabetic services might reveal inadequacies in your baseline knowledge of what services you are providing, how they are utilised or what you are achieving. This might create the opportunity to review how individuals contribute to the overall diabetic care provided – include the employed and attached staff as well as independent contractors such as the local optometrist and community pharmacist. Once you are sure of everyone's roles and responsibilities and your vision for the care that you intend to provide, you can reassess individuals' learning needs in a co-ordinated plan to match the service you will provide.

Compare your own figures for the numbers of people with diabetes with those you would expect in a practice population of your size and demographic make-up. Decide whether you need to be more pro-active in identifying new cases of diabetes, and address lack of knowledge or skills, uncaring attitudes or inadequate systems.

Compare prescribing patterns (current PACT data) between the GPs in your practice, and other practices. Look for differences and inconsistencies that may indicate learning needs.

A patient complaint may reveal learning needs for individuals or the practice organisation (e.g. a complaint from the parents of a 10-year-old boy about the delay in detecting his diabetes).

Compare your practice protocol for the management of diabetes with other recommended guidelines to reveal learning needs.

The practice nurse or health visitor might have nominated diabetes as a topic they wished to learn more about at their annual job appraisal. If no one else in the practice has expert knowledge or skills in the management of diabetes, then it will be well worth the practice facilitating the nurse to attend an in-depth course.

The practice manager may be new to the area and intend to visit other practices to learn the ropes. He or she might take a particular interest in observing how other practices run their diabetes services. This focus might justify additional time spent on practice visiting.

Patient or public input to your plan

Ask the parents who made the complaint to help you to devise better systems in the practice, or write an account of their experiences that can be used for an in-house training session.

You might ask the local representative of Diabetes UK or a patient with diabetes to attend an informal training session – in particular dealing with educating and informing patients better, and motivating patients about the prevention of risks, and the side-effects of treatment.

An open evening on diabetes that is held for patients with diabetes and their families will provide an opportunity for patients to mix with GPs, nurses, therapists, optometrists and non-clinical staff. Informal conversations during the evening should reveal learning needs and ideas for improvements.

Aims of the practice personal and professional development plan arising from the preliminary data-gathering exercise

After gathering baseline data and undertaking a preliminary learning needs assessment, you might design a practice personal and professional development plan that has a grand overarching aim, namely to develop a learning programme for all members of the practice team, attached staff and independent contractors (e.g. optometrists and community pharmacists) to enable them to provide effective management of diabetes within the available resources.

Alternatively, you might concentrate on developing particular key individuals (e.g. a GP or practice nurse or specific receptionist with lead responsibility for the clinical management or practice organisation of diabetes). They could then cascade their learning in-house to others in the practice team.

Finally, you could focus on aspects of the effective management of diabetes. For instance, you could focus on developing a learning programme for all members of the wider primary healthcare team to increase their knowledge and skills in educating and informing patients and their families about good practice in the management of diabetes. This might include learning how to motivate patients to comply with recommended management practices, avoid risks and complications, and comply with treatment.

How might you integrate the 14 components of clinical governance into your practice personal and professional development plan focusing on diabetes?

Establishing a learning culture: a multidisciplinary team might update their knowledge about reducing cardiovascular risks in people with type 2 diabetes. The practice manager could learn about setting up systems for detecting new cases of diabetes, facilitating follow-up care and encouraging compliance. The nurses and GPs could learn about risk management and better ways to motivate patients to comply with treatment.

Managing resources and services: promote close working relationships and teamwork between the practice-employed staff, independent contractors such as the optometrists and trust-employed staff such as podiatrists and district nurses.

Establishing a research and development culture: encourage practice team members to critically appraise published papers describing new findings in diabetic care, to check whether the results described are applicable to their population.

Reliable and accurate data: keep good records to enable active follow-up of any patients with diabetes who are unable to get to the surgery, such as the housebound or any others who fail to attend at regular intervals.

Evidence-based practice and policy: the practice protocol for people with different types of diabetes should be based on the best evidence for the population and local circumstances.

Confidentiality: there should be water-tight systems to prevent any information about a patient having diabetes being released without their consent. Any issues of confidentiality should be clarified before information about individuals is passed to a district register.

Health gain: good glycaemic control reduces the risk of complications from diabetes.

Coherent team: all members of the practice team should understand the roles that the attached podiatrist, optometrist and pharmacist play in providing care.

Audit and evaluation: a significant event audit of, for example, a person with diabetes becoming blind should indicate areas where further training is required, or where practice services and teamwork need to be improved.

Meaningful involvement of patients and the public: you might organise a roadshow demonstrating good diabetic care, which could be held in the surgery and attended by representatives from the voluntary sector, patients, clinicians and support staff for people with diabetes and their families. A focus group of patients with diabetes might reveal short-comings in staff knowledge and attitudes, or malfunctioning practice systems.

Health promotion: target diabetic patients with advice about their lifestyle, especially smoking.

Risk management: identifying and controlling risks is the bedrock of the management of diabetes to reduce the likelihood and extent of complications.

Accountability and performance: demonstrate that the advice and treatment which staff are providing to patients with diabetes is consistent with best practice.

Core requirements: practice staff should be competent and trained for the roles and responsibilities that are delegated to them by the GPs and practice manager.

Action plan (include the objectives above, timetabled action and expected outcomes)

Agree who is involved and the setting: as staff set out previously – specify names, posts.

Timetabled action: Start date . . .

By 3 months: preliminary data gathered and collation of baseline of providers.
- Is there a practice protocol or guide on effective management of diabetes?
- Numbers of staff; map expertise; list other providers.
- Referral patterns for routine advice and monitoring of diabetes admissions, for advice/help for complications.

- Information about the characteristics of those recorded on the practice computer as having diabetes (e.g. age groups, ethnic origins).
- Any relevant local and national priorities, and any additional associated resources for which you might apply.
- Staff discussion to report problems that limit those with diabetes of different age groups, etc., accessing services – observed problems, views and suggestions.

By 4 months: review current performance.
- Practice manager reviews operation of services and closeness of working relationships with those in other organisations and sectors who have an interest in or responsibility for diabetes.
- Clinical leads (e.g. GP, nurse) review the extent of the knowledge, skills and attitudes of the practice team with regard to routine care of those with diabetes of all types.
- Audit actual performance vs. pre-agreed criteria (e.g. with respect to referrals, education given to those with diabetes, investigations, monitoring and compliance).
- Compare performance with any or several of the 14 components of clinical governance (e.g. *health promotion would be very relevant*).

By 6 months: identify solutions and associated training needs.
- Set up new systems for access to services appropriate for those with diabetes.
- Give the practice team in-house training on important aspects of managing diabetes.
- Revise the practice protocol. Address identified gaps in care, having undertaken a search for other evidence-based protocols. Agree roles and responsibilities as a team for delivering care and services according to protocol. Certain staff attend external courses. The practice or district nurse, GP, podiatrist or optometrist provide some in-house training to other GPs and nurses, the community pharmacist or others from outside organisations with whom the practice is liaising over the issue.

By 12 months: make changes.
- Clinicians adhere to practice protocol, as shown by repeat audits; patient feedback.
- Change service times and locations so that they are more appropriate for individuals with diabetes of various age ranges and ethnic groups, having organised training to anticipate new requirements (e.g. train podiatrist to fit in with other members of the primary care team in surgery setting).

Expected outcomes: more effective prevention of diabetic complications, better patient compliance with treatment and good lifestyle habits, tighter glucose control, fewer patients with diabetes being lost to follow-up.

How does your practice personal and professional development plan tie in with your other strategic plans?

The practice's business plan and the PCO's Primary Care Investment Plan might both prioritise achieving more effective management of diabetes. Diabetes is a priority in the health improvement programme. The practice personal and professional development plan that focuses on diabetes would complement those strategic plans.

What additional resources will you require to execute your plan and from where do you hope to obtain them?

The practice might pay for the course fees of any member of staff undertaking training that fulfils a priority need of the practice.

You may be able to justify an application for additional resources to your PCO or health authority or local NHS trust with your preliminary learning and health needs assessments, tapping into the district or national strategic priorities.

If a member of staff is undertaking the training on behalf of the practice, you should try to arrange for the training to be undertaken in paid time. Any learning that is cascaded to other members of the practice team as part of the practice personal and professional development plan should also be undertaken in paid time and during working hours whenever possible.

How will you evaluate your practice personal and professional development plan?

You should be able to select methods of evaluation from the range of methods suggested for assessing learning needs in the first section of this book. The most appropriate methods will depend on what specific aims you set for your practice personal and professional development plan. For example, if your main aim is to achieve the best possible glucose control in people with diabetes, you might evaluate this by monitoring HbA_{1c} levels. However, if your aim is to improve the levels and appropriateness of education and information for people with diabetes, you might evaluate your achievements by asking the patients themselves – by a simple test of knowledge, focus-group discussion of experiences, monitoring changes in patient behaviour, etc.

The practice manager and clinical lead for diabetes (e.g. the GP or practice nurse) might plan the evaluation together and delegate the collection of data to a receptionist.

How will you know when you have achieved your objectives?

Usually this will be by comparing the outcomes of your programme with baseline data. However, it might also be determined by looking at patients' compliance with recommended practice, or their levels of self-confidence in managing their diabetic condition (asking and attending for help at appropriate times).

How will you disseminate the learning from the plan to the rest of the practice team and patients? How will you sustain the new knowledge and skills?

You might write about it in a practice newsletter. Let all the staff know at practice meetings what progress has been made. You might want to describe your success at a PCG meeting.

Pass on your skills and knowledge to others as required, and review your protocol at set intervals in order to incorporate new information.

How will you handle new learning requirements as they crop up?

The practice manager might run audits at intervals and feed the results back to a practice meeting mid-way through the time period of the practice personal and professional development plan, when there is time to revise the activities.

Record of practice team learning about Diabetes

You would add the date, length of time spent, etc., for each learning activity

	Activity 1 – revise practice protocol	Activity 2 – update patient education	Activity 3 – identification of new diabetics	Activity 4 – preventing complications of diabetes
In-house formal learning	Practice team discussion around roles and responsibilities of various members to fulfil protocol, including district nurses, podiatrist and optometrist	A pharmaceutical representative shows a non-promotional video on educating people with diabetes, which is watched by GPs, nurses and the community pharmacist	GP and nurse with new ideas on targeting and detection (*see below*) share their ideas with the rest of the practice team during practice discussion of diabetic protocol (*see Activity 1*)	Hospital specialist input to follow-up practice team discussion when changes to practice protocol are reviewed, with any changes in HBA_{1c} levels resulting
External courses	GP lead on diabetes attends two-day continuing medical education course on diabetes at regional centre			Practice nurse attends half-day course on health promotion and motivating patients. She extrapolates this learning to diabetes.
Informal and personal	Practice nurse searches for examples of best practice on Medline at home. Practice manager rings up other practices to ask other practice managers if they have protocols, and discusses differences	After watching the video, the practice manager brings in all of the diabetic literature and audio-visual aids available. The team then sorts them according to criteria already set from a previous initiative on asthma	A GP attending a two-day external course and a practice nurse attending a local practice nurse group meeting pick up tips for targeted screening and being more alert to the possibility of diabetes	Practice team members all learn from talking to patients with diabetes in the course of their daily work how to make more impact with recommendations for a healthier lifestyle
Qualifications and/or experience gained	GP receives accreditation for two-day course that can be put towards a university certificate in health practice			Practice nurse attendance at a half-day course is recorded in her own reflective portfolio for discussion with her clinical supervisor

References

1 NHS Executive (2001) *National Service Framework for Diabetes.* Department of Health, London.
2 NHS Executive (2000) *The NHS Plan.* NHS Executive, London.
3 Wakley G, Chambers R and Field S (2000) *Continuing Professional Development: making it happen.* Radcliffe Medical Press, Oxford.
4 World Health Organization (1999) *Definition, Diagnosis and Classification of Diabetes Mellitus and its Complications. Part 1. Diagnosis and classification of diabetes mellitus.* World Health Organization, Geneva.
5 Williams R and Farrar H (2001) Diabetes mellitus. In: *Health Needs Assessment Series: the epidemiologically based needs assessment reviews.* Radcliffe Medical Press, Oxford. (Available online at http:// hcna.radcliffe-online.com/diabframe.htm)
6 Chambers R and Wakley G (2000) *Making Clinical Governance Work for You.* Radcliffe Medical Press, Oxford.
7 Commission for Health Improvement (2000) *Clinical Governance Reviews: an overview.* Commission for Health Improvement, London.
8 Jachuck S (2000) Management of diabetes mellitus in general practice. *Cardiol Gen Pract.* **7**: 429–32.
9 Dunning M, Abi-Aad G, Gilbert D *et al.* (1999) *Experience, Evidence and Everyday Practice.* King's Fund, London.
10 Chambers R (2000) *Involving Patients and the Public: how to do it better.* Radcliffe Medical Press, Oxford.
11 Clinical Standards Advisory Group (1994) *Report on Standards of Clinical Care for People with Diabetes.* HMSO, London.
12 Department of Health (1997) Report of the review of patient-identifiable information. In: *The Caldicott Committee Report.* Department of Health, London.
13 Donald P (2000) Promoting local ownership of guidelines. *Guidelines Pract.* **3**: 17.
14 Diabetes Control and Complications Trial (DCCT) Research Group (1993) The effect of intensive treatment of diabetes on the development and progression of long-term complications in insulin-dependent diabetes mellitus. *NEJM.* **329**: 977–86.
15 United Kingdom Prospective Diabetes Study (UKPDS) Group (1998) Intensive blood-glucose control with sulphonylureas or insulin compared

with conventional treatment and risk of complications in patients with type 2 diabetes (UKPDS 33). *Lancet.* **352:** 837–53.

16 Muir Gray JA (1997) *Evidence-Based Healthcare.* Churchill Livingstone, Edinburgh.

17 Barton S (ed.) (2000) *Clinical Evidence. Issue 4.* BMJ Publishing Group, London.

18 Scottish Intercollegiate Guidelines Network (1997) *Management of Diabetic Renal Disease. National clinical guideline for Scotland.* Scottish Intercollegiate Guidelines Network, Edinburgh.

19 Scottish Intercollegiate Guidelines Network (1997) *Management of Diabetic Foot Disease. National clinical guideline for Scotland.* Scottish Intercollegiate Guidelines Network, Edinburgh.

20 Scottish Intercollegiate Guidelines Network (1998) *Prevention of Visual Impairment. National clinical guideline for Scotland.* Scottish Intercollegiate Guidelines Network, Edinburgh.

21 Scottish Intercollegiate Guidelines Network (1996) *Management of Diabetes in Pregnancy. National clinical guideline for Scotland.* Scottish Intercollegiate Guidelines Network, Edinburgh.

22 Scottish Intercollegiate Guidelines Network (1997) *Management of Diabetic Cardiovascular Disease. National clinical guideline for Scotland.* Scottish Intercollegiate Guidelines Network, Edinburgh.

23 Melville A (2000) Complications of diabetes: renal disease and promotion of self-management. *Effect Health Care Bull.* **6:** 1–12.

24 Holden P (2000) GP's diabetes clinic has improved patient care. *Pulse.* **19 August:** 32–5.

25 James M, Turner DA, Broadbent DM *et al.* (2000) Cost-effectiveness analysis of screening for sight-threatening diabetic eye disease. *BMJ.* **320:** 1627–31.

26 NHS Centre for Reviews and Dissemination (1999) Complications of diabetes: screening for retinopathy; management of foot ulcers. *Effect Health Care Bull.* **5:** 1–12.

27 Mohanna K and Chambers R (2001) *Risk Matters in Healthcare: communicating, explaining and managing risk.* Radcliffe Medical Press, Oxford.

28 Watkins P (1998) *ABC of Diabetes.* BMJ Publishing Group, London.

29 Diabetes UK (2000) *Position Statement. New diagnostic criteria for diabetes.* Diabetes UK (previously British Diabetic Association), London.

30 Bingley P, Douek I, Rogers C *et al.* (2000) Influence of maternal age at delivery and birth order on risk of type 1 diabetes in childhood: prospective population-based family study. *BMJ.* **321:** 420–4.

31 King's Fund Policy Institute (1996) *Counting the Cost: the real impact of non-insulin-dependent diabetes.* King's Fund, London.

32 Bennett N, Dodd T, Flatley J *et al.* (1993) *Health Survey for England. Social Survey Division of Population Censuses and Surveys.* HMSO, London.

33 Calman K (1998) *On the State of the Public Health.* The Annual Report of

the Chief Medical Officer of the Department of Health for the year 1997. The Stationery Office, London.

34 Diabetes UK (2000) *Diabetes in the UK – the missing million*. Diabetes UK (previously British Diabetic Association), London.

35 Gray A, Raikou M, McGuire A *et al.* (UKPDS Group) (2000) Cost-effectiveness of an intensive blood glucose control policy in patients with type 2 diabetes: economic analysis alongside randomised control trial (UKPDS 41). *BMJ.* **320**: 1373–8.

36 Expert Committee on the Diagnosis and Classification of Diabetes Mellitus (1997) Report of the Expert Committee on the Diagnosis and Classification of Diabetes Mellitus. *Diabetes Care.* **20**: 1183–97.

37 Sackett DL and Holland WW (1975) Controversy in the detection of disease. *Lancet.* **2**: 357–9.

38 Foord-Kelsey G (ed.) (2001) *Guidelines*. Medendium Group, Berkhamsted.

39 Broadbent D (2000) Diabetic eye disease: how can it be prevented? *Practitioner.* **244**: 696–701.

40 Donnelly R, Emslie-Smith AM, Gardner ID *et al.* (2000) Vascular complications of diabetes. *BMJ.* **320**: 1062–66.

41 Brown G, Brown M, Sharma S *et al.* (2000) Quality of life associated with diabetes mellitus in an adult population. *J Diabetes Complicat.* **14**: 18–24.

42 Albert KG (1992) Good control or a happy life? In: I Lewin and C Seymour (eds) *Current Themes in Diabetes Care*. Royal College of Physicians, London.

43 Stratton IM, Adler AI, Neil AW *et al.* (UKPDS Group) (2000) Association of glycaemia with macrovascular and microvascular complications of type 2 diabetes (UKPDS 35): prospective observational study. *BMJ.* **321**: 405–12.

44 Bhattacharya S (2000) Study highlights lipids link to diabetes-related deaths (preliminary report). *Pulse.* **1 July**: 27.

45 Chandalia M, Garg A, Lutjohann D *et al.* (2000) Beneficial effects of high dietary fiber intake in patients with type 2 diabetes mellitus. *NEJM.* **342**: 1392–8.

46 Jones JM, Lawson ML, Daneman D *et al.* (2000) Eating disorders in adolescent females with and without type 1 diabetes: cross-sectional study. *BMJ.* **320**: 1563–6.

47 Hutchinson A, McIntosh A, Feder G *et al.* (2000) *Clinical Guidelines for Type 2 Diabetes. Prevention and management of foot problems*. Royal College of General Practitioners, London.

48 White S, Nicholson M and Hering B (2000) Can islet-cell transplantation treat diabetes? *BMJ.* **321**: 651–2.

49 Wood D, Durrington P, Poulter N *et al.* (1998) Joint British recommendations on prevention of coronary heart disease in clinical practice. *Heart.* **80 (Supplement 2)**: S1–29.

50 Guidelines Working Group (2000) Guidelines – reducing the risk of CHD in diabetic patients. *Br J Cardiol.* **7**: 290–2.

51 Mehta D (ed.) (2000) *British National Formulary. Issue 40.* British Medical Association and the Royal Pharmaceutical Society of Great Britain, London.

52 Collier J (ed.) (1999) Reducing long-term complications of type 2 diabetes. *Drug Ther Bull.* **37**: 84–7.

53 Adler A, Stratton I, Neil HA *et al.* (2000) Association of systolic blood pressure with macrovascular and microvascular complications of type 2 diabetes (UKPDS 36): prospective observational study. *BMJ.* **321**: 412–9.

54 UK Prospective Diabetes Study Group (1998) Tight blood pressure control and risk of macrovascular and microvascular complications in type 2 diabetes (UKPDS 38). *BMJ.* **317**: 703–12.

55 Gress T, Nieto J, Shahar E *et al.* (2000) Hypertension and antihypertensive therapy as risk factors for type 2 diabetes mellitus. *NEJM.* **342**: 905–12.

56 Fox C and MacKinnon M (1999) *Vital Diabetes.* Class Heath, London.

57 Heart Outcomes Prevention Evaluation Study Investigators (2000) Effects of ramipril on cardiovascular and microvascular outcomes in people with diabetes mellitus: results of the HOPE and MICRO-HOPE substudy. *Lancet.* **355**: 253–9.

58 UK Prospective Diabetes Study Group (1998) Effect of intensive blood-glucose control with metformin on complications in overweight patients with type 2 diabetes (UKPDS 34). *Lancet.* **352**: 854–65.

59 Morris A (2000) *First UK Population-Based Study Reveals Two-Thirds of Patients With Type 2 Diabetes Fail to Adhere to Prescribed Drug Programmes.* University of Dundee, Tayside.

60 National Institute for Clinical Excellence (2000) *Guidance on Rosiglitazone for Type 2 Diabetes Mellitus.* National Institute for Clinical Excellence, London.

61 Flanagan DEH, Holt H and Cavan D (2000) Insulin treatment in type 2 diabetes – who benefits? *Diabet Med.* **17**: 84 (abstract).

62 Boulton A (2000) Management of diabetic peripheral neuropathy. *Prescrib J.* **40**: 107–12.

63 Lovell HG (1999) *Are Angiotensin-Converting Enzyme Inhibitors Useful for Normotensive Diabetic Patients with Microalbuminuria?* (Cochrane Review). The Cochrane Library, Oxford.

64 Coster S, Gulliford MC, Seed PT *et al.* (2000) Monitoring blood glucose control in diabetes mellitus: a systematic review. *Health Technol Assess.* **4**: 1–95.

65 Greenhalgh PM (1994) *Shared Care for Diabetes. A systematic review.* Occasional Paper 67. Royal College of General Practitioners, London.

66 Pennington J and Taylor LJ (2000) A diabetes knowledge assessment tool to improve provision of patient education. *Diabet Med.* **17** (**Supplement 1**): 43 (abstract).

67 World Health Organization (1995) *Diabetes Care and Research in Europe:*

the Saint Vincent Declaration action programme. Implementation document. WHO, Copenhagen.

68 Gormley DA and Baksi AK (2000) Do people with diabetes desire a role in diabetes treatment decisions? *Diabet Med.* **17 (Supplement 1)**: 41 (abstract).

69 British Diabetic Association (1992) *Diabetes Care. What you should expect.* British Diabetic Association (now Diabetes UK), London.

70 O'Brien SV and Hardy KJ (2000) Integrated care pathway-driven diabetes education associated with highly significant improvements in diabetes knowledge, diabetes well-being and HbA$_{1c}$. *Diabet Med.* **17 (Supplement 1)**: 19 (abstract).

71 Carroll C, Naylor E, Marsden P *et al.* (2000) Cardiovascular risk perception in patients with type 2 diabetes. *Diabet Med.* **17 (Supplement 1)**: 19 (abstract).

72 Browne D, Avery L, Turner B *et al.* (2000) What do patients with diabetes know about their tablets? *Diabet Med.* **17**: 528–31.

73 Carroll C, Naylor E, Marsden P *et al.* (2000) Cardiovascular risk perception in patients with type 2 diabetes. *Diabet Med.* **17 (Supplement 1)**: 19 (abstract).

74 Scottish Intercollegiate Guidelines Network (1996) *Report on Good Practice in the Care of Children and Young People with Diabetes.* Scottish Intercollegiate Guidelines Network, Edinburgh.

75 Drury H (2000) Growing up with diabetes. *Pulse.* **60**: 71.

76 Donnan PT, MacDonald TM and Morris AD (2000) Adherence to prescribed medication for patients with type 2 diabetes: a population study. *Diabet Med.* **17 (Supplement 1)**: 2.

77 Gadsby R (2000) Improving concordance in type 2 diabetes. *Prescrib Suppl.* 3–6.

78 McKinnon M (2000) The role of the nurse. *Prescrib Suppl.* 7.

79 Pierce M, Agarwal G and Ridout D (2000) A survey of diabetes care in general practice in England and Wales. *Br J Gen Pract.* **50**: 542–5.

80 Lockyer M (2000) Shared care is the key to success of primary care diabetes clinic. *Guidelines Pract.* **3**: 41–9.

81 Thomson M, Frost J and Gornall R (2000) Implementation of guidelines for the assessment of the diabetic foot in the primary care setting. *Diabet Med.* **17 (Supplement 1)**: 80 (abstract).

82 Walker A, Davies S and Neary R (2000) *Microalbuminuria Screening.* Circular letter to all general practitioners in North Staffordshire. Department of Endocrinology and Diabetes Mellitus, City General Hospital, Stoke-on-Trent.

83 Williams E, Beer J and Marouf ES (2000) Diabetes care in nursing and residential homes. *Diabet Med.* **17 (Supplement 1)**: 21 (abstract).

84 Audit Commission (2000) *Testing Times. A review of diabetes services in England and Wales.* Audit Commission, London.

85 Prasad S (2000) Creating a district diabetes register: input from primary and secondary care is necessary for success. *Br J Gen Pract.* **50**: 826 (letter).

86 Hardy KJ and O'Brien SV (2000) Integrated care pathway associated with reduction in diabetes non-attenders from 19% to 1%. *Diabet Med.* **17 (Supplement 1)**: 19 (abstract).

87 Boyle DIR, Brennan GM, Devers MC *et al.* (2000) An online Web-based educational and clinical resource for the management of patients with diabetes. *Diabet Med.* **17 (Supplement 1)**: 11 (abstract).

88 British Diabetic Association (1999) *Recommendations for the Structure of Specialist Diabetes Care Services.* British Diabetic Association (now Diabetes UK), London.

89 British Diabetic Association (1998) *Diabetes Centres in the United Kingdom. Results of a survey of UK diabetes centres.* British Diabetic Association (now Diabetes UK), London.

Sources of help

Websites for guidelines and information

Agency for Healthcare Research and Quality	http://www.ahcpr.gov
Bandolier	http://ebandolier.com
Canadian Medical Association	http://www.cma.ca/cpgs/
Centres for Health Evidence	www.cche.net/principles/content_all.asp
Cochrane Collaboration	http://www.cochrane.org
Diabetes UK	http://www.diabetes.org.uk
*e*Guidelines	http://www.eguidelines.co.uk
General Medical Council	http://www.gmc-uk.org
Guideline Project	http://www.ihs.ox.ac.uk/guidelines/
HoN (Health on the Net)	http://www.hon.ch
Medline	http://www.omni.ac.uk/medline
New Zealand Guidelines Group	http://www.nzgg.org.nz
NLM Health Services (Technology Assessment)	http://www.nlm.nih.gov
North of England Evidence-Based Guidelines	http://www.ncl.ac.uk/~ncenthsr/publicn/publicn.htm
OMNI (Organising Medical Networked Information)	http://www.omni.ac.uk
PRODIGY	http://www.prodigy.nhs.uk
Radcliffe Online	www.primarycareonline.co.uk
Scottish Intercollegiate Network Guidelines (SIGN)	http://www.sign.ac.uk
Significant Event Audit	http://latis.ex.ac.uk/sigevent/
St George's Health Care Evaluation Unit	http://www.sghms.ac.uk/depts/phs/hceu/nhsguide.htm
UK Health Centre	http://www.healthcentre.org.uk/hc/library/guidelines.htm
WISDOM Centre	http://www.wisdomnet.co.uk

Resources for people with diabetes

Diabetes UK Careline. Tel: 020 7636 6112; e-mail: <u>careline@diabetes.org.uk</u>

Diabetes UK catalogue of books, diet and cookery booklets, emergency identity cards, and *Guidelines for Diagnosing and Classifying Diabetes, June 2000.* All from Diabetes UK, 10 Queen Anne Street, London W1M 0BD. Tel: 020 7462 2791 or 0800 585 088, or e-mail <u>customerservice@diabetes.org.uk</u>

Living with Diabetes and the Coeliac Condition. Published by Nutricia Dietary Care, Newmarket Avenue, White Horse Business Park, Trowbridge, Wiltshire BA14 0XQ, in association with Diabetes UK.

MedicAlert, 12 Bridge Wharf, 156 Caledonian Road, London N1 9UU.

Medical Aspects of Fitness to Drive. Driver and Vehicle Licensing Agency, Swansea SA9 1AB.

Understanding diabetes. Published by Family Doctor Publications, 10 Butchers Row, Banbury, Oxon OX16 8JH. Tel: 01295 276627; e-mail: <u>familydoctor@btinternet.com</u> in association with the British Medical Association.

Index